Double Crossed

A Review of the Most Extreme Exercise Program

By Dr. Sean M. Wells
PT, DPT, OCS, ATC/L, CSCS, NSCA-CPT

Printed in the United States of America

First Edition, June 2014
Second Edition, November 2014

ISBN 978-0-9904358-2-2; E-pub ISBN 978-0-9904358-3-9

Wells Physical Therapy, LLC
1575 Pine Ridge Road Ste. 20
Naples, FL 34109

www.double-crossed.com

Acknowledgments

To Rebecca for her integrity, faithfulness, and love;
To Logan – the little agent of change.

Thank you to my friends and family – I swear I am not a hermit!

David Lee, thank you for your amazing work with the layout of this book.
Sonja Putsay, thank you for the help with the images.

To my mentors: Joel, John, Dave, and Amy – you inspire me.

To my clients and students: you are my drive to learn more.

About the Author

Dr. Sean M. Wells, PT, DPT, OCS, ATC/L, CSCS, NSCA-CPT

Dr. Sean Wells has a passion for health, sports medicine and evidence-based practice. He serves clientele from professional and Division I athletes to top Fortune 500 company executives.

Dr. Sean Wells holds a Doctorate of Physical Therapy, is a Licensed Athletic Trainer as well as a Certified Strength and Conditioning Specialist and Personal Trainer. Sean is a member of the American Physical Therapy Association and The National Strength and Conditioning Association. He has taught sports medicine and exercise physiology at both the graduate and undergraduate levels. He has published in national and international journals and holds symposiums on aging, orthopedics, and wound care. Dr. Wells is a contributing author to Muscle and Fitness and E'Bella Magazine, as well as Livestrong.com. He is active with research in long-term stroke rehab, osteoporosis cases, and aging models.

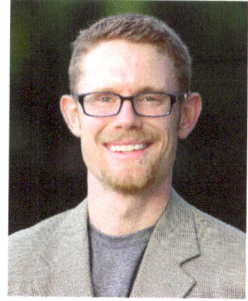

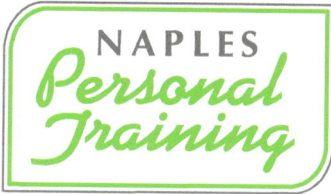

NAPLES *Personal Training*

Dr. Sean Wells is the owner and operator of Naples Personal Training located in Naples, FL. His center is renowned for its excellence in fitness and rehabilitation. He enjoys training with his wife, adventuring to the beach with his son, and helping others live healthy lifestyles.

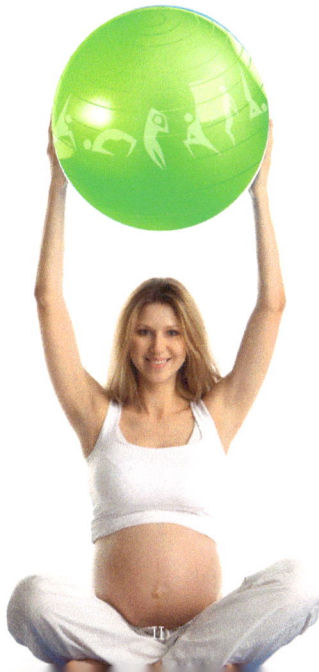

Preface

I originally published this book in June 2014 with the intent of educating the masses of the risk of a fast-growing extreme exercise program. In my first edition I cited current research, anecdotal evidence, and provided scientific theory as to how a specific extreme exercise program could seriously harm you. Can this program help you? Sure. You can lose weight, gain muscle mass, but most exercise specialists across the world are asking: at what cost? I am happy to say it only took 4 months for my book to scare this company's legal and business team into finding a way to stop me.

I cannot name the name of the exercise program for their legal team will likely shut down my printing company on grounds of trademark infringement as they did in October 2014. If you are picking up this book and are still unsure of the company's name, I am positive you can infer it from the title "Double-Crossed." If you still are struggling at identifying this extreme exercise program continue reading and search the sources I have provided below. Throughout the book you will see my citation of "X-Company." This will be my only means of addressing this extreme exercise program without infringing on their trademark rights.

After X-Company used a false trademark infringement to shut my book down, I realized the opportunity for me to add additional data and publications to my book. As such, you will find even more current research and up-to-date "news." This shows my dedication to remaining current with the literature and evidence.

Probably the key purpose of this second edition is to ensure I can enact my freedom of speech – a God given right of all Americans. We all should be able to freely publish a book, whether positive or negative, about another's concept or product. This stems further discussion, debate, and potential progress. Doing so can also provide further divide, which is something I am not interested in creating.

During the four months of open publication I received much feedback. Some of the positive feedback centered on the need for more regulation in the fitness industry and how my book covered multiple areas of this extreme exercise program. I received feedback from those participating in X-Company's exercise program, some of whom are my friends. Several agreed that the extreme exercise program was not "quite-right for everyone" or was a "good addition to a traditional exercise program." They saw major limitations in the exercise program, knew it could be better, and even cited that it "grew out proportion from how it was meant to be started." A significant portion of those exercising in X-Company's program provided little meaningful discussion or feedback. Again, the purpose of this book was to not drive a further wedge between "traditional" exercise and X-Company's exercise – it was to start the discussion for a better future for everyone.

I hope you enjoy this second edition and that it paints a path for lifelong health and safe exercising for you and your family.

Table of Contents

Introduction

X-Company is a global phenomenon. Some may call it a workout, a way of life, a fad, or even a cult. Regardless of what you call it, each year nearly 1 million people participate in X-Company in some capacity. The entity X-Company has grown at a blazing rate with over ten thousand centers in eleven years.

Growth and interest in an exercise-related activity is fabulous news for many Western countries that are struggling with obesity and chronic health issues. Countless research articles and scientists have pointed to the benefits of physical activity and exercise. However, most if not all of these esteemed researchers have examined traditional exercise modes and routines, not X-Company. Thousands of subjects over the course of several decades have been tested, measured, and progressed on many of the traditional exercise methods within the scientific literature. Is X-Company too young to be held equivalent to these traditional exercise methods? Have its methods and safety been properly vetted? As an exercise specialist and researcher, I believe, based on research and sound exercise theories, that X-Company is not the remedy for our health crisis. Sure, you might lose weight and gain strength doing X-Company—but at what cost?

Here is the forewarning: if you are an X-Company enthusiast, this book will make you uncomfortable. It will explain how the X-Company concept started and propagated, criticize the safety aspects of X-Company, and analyze several of the movements and progressions involved. This book serves a purpose to educate and help you analyze the risks of X-Company so you can make an informed choice. Furthermore, I hope that this book will increase the awareness of X-Company's problems so that we can work toward making a necessary positive change in the professions of exercise and rehabilitation. This book will also provide you with simple tips on how to choose a facility, personal trainer, and basic exercise principles before you begin or continue your exercise journey. Exercise is a lifelong process: it offers an endless number of benefits, often with little cost. I hope that you too can see the beauty in lifelong exercise. After you read this book, I know you will find the best exercise that meets your needs so you can move forward, armed with knowledge, to educate others about the risks of X-Company.

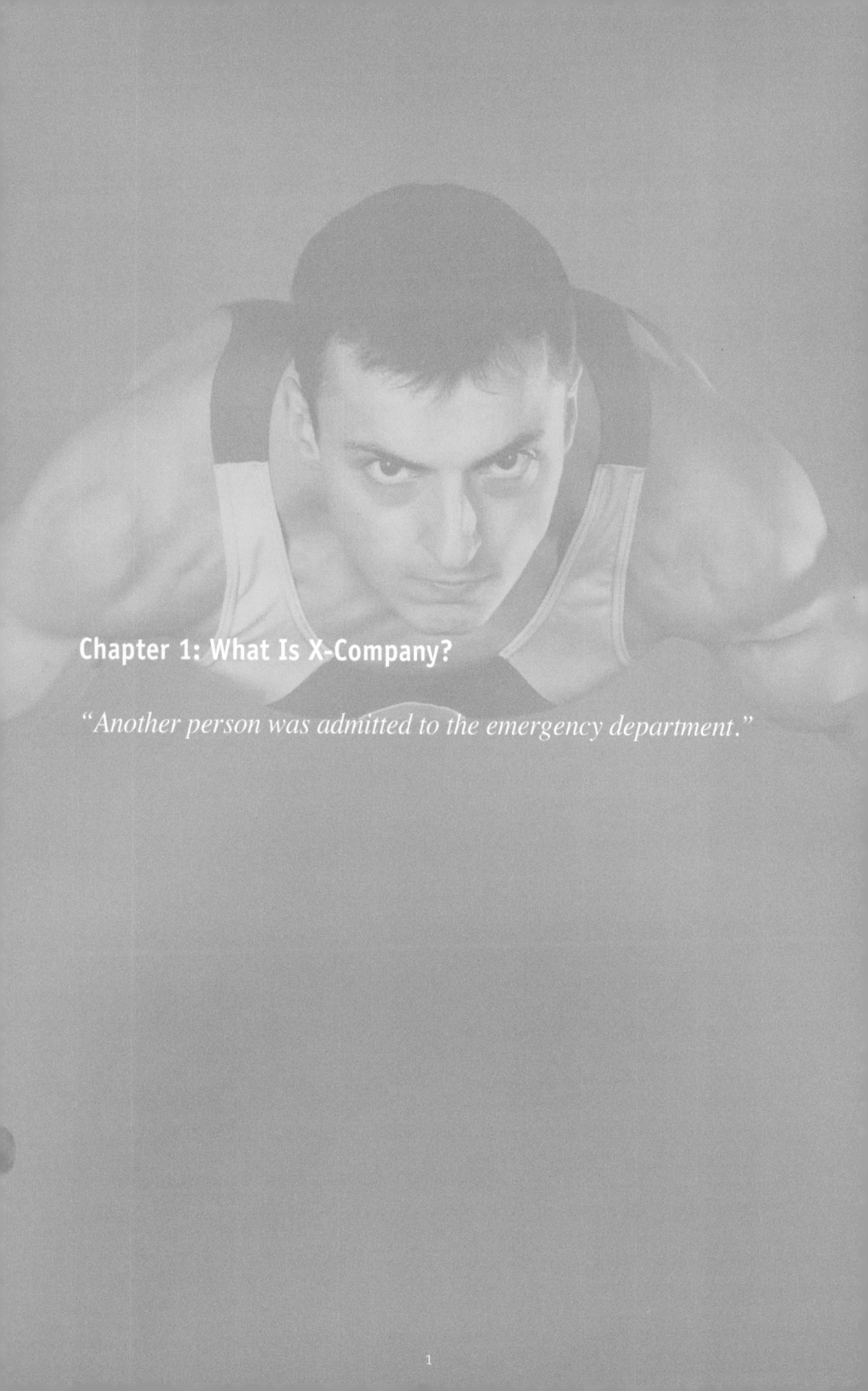

Chapter 1: What Is X-Company?

"Another person was admitted to the emergency department."

If you are wavering on joining an X-Company gym or at least trying a session, consider what Greg Glassman, the founder of X-Company, has to tell you from his interview with the New York Times: "If you find the notion of falling off the rings and breaking your neck so foreign to you, then we don't want you in our ranks."

At this point, alarms should be ringing in your head. Three options exist if the founder of an exercise organization does not want you because you are scared of injuring yourself while engaged in his business of exercise:

1. The exercise organization lacks accreditation, **education,** and professional judgment.

2. You have failed to do your research on the best organization for long-term health - and skill-related fitness.

3. He does not care about your well-being.

Read this book to understand why I make such a strong statement in point one. You will eliminate point two from your choices. And, after examining the facts, you can form your own opinion about point three.

From Kevin Ogar, the X-Company trainer who severed his spinal cord during an X-Company competition, to the hundreds of people who have been hospitalized for life-threatening muscle breakdown called rhabdo, this book is about real people and an exercise program that goes too far.

The Journey

As I walk into the Human Performance Lab at Florida Gulf Coast University, the lab director, Dr. Dennis Hunt, turns to me and remarks, "Another person was admitted to the emergency department."

Dr. Hunt was counting the number of admissions to the local emergency department for rhabdomyolysis due to X-Company training. Although we jokingly kept a "count" of the admissions, we both knew that X-Company was having a serious impact on our community members. All jokes aside, rhabdomyolysis, commonly referred to as "Uncle Rhabdo" by X-Company exercisers, is a serious and potentially deadly medical condition. Rhabdomyolysis involves a full-body breakdown of proteins, the shutting down of the kidneys, and potential heart arrhythmias. No one was joking when we heard that at least three of our students on campus had been admitted to the hospital with this dangerous condition that year.

As professors in the Exercise Science Program, we both share a passion for exercise and had conducted several research studies examining how the human body responds to exercise. Dr. Hunt has spent much of his last twenty years in academia examining the effects of weight training. I found a unique interest in sports medicine and orthopedics. As such, we follow trends, read intriguing journal articles, speak at national conferences, and keep in contact with the local community of fitness and rehab specialists. One thing we both noted was that X-Company was on the rise in both South Florida and the rest of the country. Another thing we realized is that we did not know enough about it to properly educate our students. This became strikingly apparent after I assigned a student a project.

In teaching a sports medicine injury prevention course in 2012, I included what I call a "topic summary." Students were to choose a topic of interest and research how an injury could be treated and prevented. The research needed to be evidenced based and peer reviewed—I had educated them on Sackett's hierarchy of evidence (http://www.cebm.net/), which states that certain research studies are higher levels of evidence than others. The level of research is based on the number of participants, blinding, study design, and other factors. Based on this level of evidence, exercise specialists can make sound, scientific decisions for their clients.

I had one student who was very interested in exercise-induced rhabdo. He visited me in my office and we discussed how exercise scientists had tackled this topic; it was already in his textbook. So I tasked this excelling student to answer the question, what is the prevalence of rhabdomyolysis in X-Company training? He showed excitement to be researching something so contemporary and important to our field.

Several weeks later I receive an email: "Dr. Wells, I cannot find any research articles on this topic. I am afraid I may not be able to complete the assignment." I was a bit dismayed at first, but I encouraged him to continue searching. I provided the names of several other major exercise and medical research databases, such as PEDro, CINAHL, and PubMed. I thought the new guidance would allow him to find at least one article. However, to my surprise, I was dead wrong.

He returned to my office the following week with nothing to show. He reported to me that the only sources available were "websites" and "blogs." He found no professional, peer-reviewed scientific articles related to rhabdo and X-Company.

Hence the journey to learn about CrossFit began…

What Is X-Company? Defining the Indefinable

Defining X-Company was challenging. After my student and I found nothing related to rhabdo and X-Company in the research databases, I continued my search online and found several Internet-based resources. I did find one scientific peer-reviewed article on X-Company, but the study was small and focused on a diet program—it had little information on X-Company's details, program, and safety.

Another study, published in November of 2013 found a significant decrease in percent body fat and a significant increase in the exerciser's oxygen utilization during exercise. The positives of this study are quickly diminished when you examine that the study lacked a control and a comparison group (e.g. a group of people doing traditional exercises). Moreover, this study became quite a quagmire for both X-Company and the publisher, the National Strength and Conditioning Association (NSCA). During the follow up period 11 of the 43 X-Company exercisers did not return for follow-up testing. The authors of the study have come forward stating that the exercisers had "injuries." Meanwhile, X-Company has come forward stating that they were not injured and the authors did not provide follow-up calls. The study was meant to blind the authors from the exercising participants, which would support X-Company's statement; perhaps the legal system will find a resolution to this issue.

The majority of the detailed information I found was from X-Company's website, the foundational and official website of X-Company Inc. X-Company began in 2003 in Santa Cruz, California. An overweight man by the name of Greg Glassman established X-Company via a blog online. He also founded two gyms in the Santa Cruz area.

The intentions of establishing the blog were far more important to Greg Glassman. He had a vision of utilizing the blog to scale his business beyond any traditional marketing concept. Many in the fitness industry were skeptical initially. Today, many in the fitness industry have been stunned at X-Company's expansion through a blog.

For some of you that may not be familiar with a blog, it is basically a website that allows people to write and post their ideas. A supervising administrator can "oversee" the discussions. Unlike chat rooms, these discussions are usually permanent fixtures of the website (unless removed by the administrator).

By 2004 to 2005, Glassman's blog blossomed and his plan to expand was in full motion. Many individuals who were training with X-Company would post suggested exercises, diet plans, and lifestyle suggestions to the blog—a sort of community wellness-sharing center. Many of these people in the early days were performing X-Company at non-X-Company gyms, wellness centers, and outdoor areas. The concept of X-Company was out on the World Wide Web; however, the facilities, equipment, and X-Company trainers had not yet made it nationwide. After 2005, America began seeing X-Company facilities popping up in large numbers. This trend would continue exponentially over the next six years.

I recall my first exposure to the X-Company blog while visiting a Navy SEAL friend in San Diego in 2009. I was in town for a national physical therapy conference, and my friend was kind enough to allow me to stay with him. While enjoying time together, we discussed his exercise routine and some of his struggles with musculoskeletal pains. He remarked that he had found a "new" routine on a blog that updated every day, exposing him to new training tips and diets. He pulled the blog up on his computer for us to review; I was excited to see such a great commitment to functional training and higher-intensity exercise. Little did I know the target market for these activities would eventually not be Navy SEALs or football players, but potentially my sixty-five-year-old mother with an arthritic hip.

The official website defines X-Company as "…many things. Primarily, it's a fitness regimen developed by Coach Greg Glassman over several decades. He was the first person in history to define fitness in a meaningful, measurable way (increased work capacity across broad time and modal domains). X-Company itself is defined as that which optimizes fitness (constantly varied functional movements performed at relatively high intensity). X-Company is also the community that spontaneously arises when people do these workouts together. In fact, the communal aspect of X-Company is a key component of why it's so effective."

Even a nonexercising person should be able to look at this definition and sense something is not completely accurate. Certainly as an exercise expert, I had my doubts and a litany of questions. For instance, how could one state he is the first person in history to define fitness in a meaningful way? Decades before X-Company was founded, the American College of Sports Medicine (ACSM) clearly defined the components of health-related fitness and continues to provide evolving national standards for these components. The components are cardiorespiratory endurance (e.g., how long you can walk or bike), muscular strength (e.g., how much weight you can lift or press), muscular endurance (e.g., how many times you can lift or move), and muscular flexibly (ability for your joints to move through an arc of motion). The components of health-related fitness are evolving as professionals continue to discuss including other factors of physical functioning, such as balance. Furthermore, the ACSM publishes guidelines that are updated frequently on how to measure fitness using tests. Certified health-care providers can easily provide these assessments, which then often guide how much exercise should be done. With the "Exercise is Medicine" initiative growing stronger, professionals around the globe in the major exercise associations are embracing the standardization of fitness assessment with proper exercise prescription (http://exerciseismedicine.org/fitpros.htm). The standardization of fitness is analogous to a physician writing a prescription for a drug after he or she has assessed you. In this example, exercise science has followed the scientific method similar to medicine: hypothesize, test/measure, assess, and treat. It appears that Glassman's X-Company concept is not the first to define fitness. X-Company goes further stating they claim fame to defining the "sport" of fitness. But what does this mean, and how can you "own" fitness?

Looking at the technical exercise components of X-Company's definition, it is obvious that X-Company provides constantly varied functional movements at high intensity, which is unique to X-Company. Functional movements are considered movements that are useful in everyday tasks or activity-related movements. An example would be a squat exercise with the purpose of improving your ability to rise from a soft chair. Functional movements have a vital role in exercise and rehabilitation; however, when not prescribed correctly or overused, functional exercises can be detrimental. From a simplistic standpoint, X-Company provides very intense, full-body exercises, typically done in a nontraditional exercise setting called a "box." The people, the equipment, and the community inside this "box" are far different than what you may expect. More will be discussed later on the exercise methods, facilities, and personalities within X-Company.

The X-Company.com website continues to explain that trainers specialize in "not specializing," which seems profoundly counterintuitive. Furthermore, it contradicts the X-Company trainers' belief of practicality that is taught in their educational seminars. X-Company stresses to their new trainers that exercises must be practical; otherwise they should not be used in a workout. I think specializing in a field as diverse as fitness and exercise is extremely practical. In addition, specialization makes you stand out from the pack of other trainers. X-Company indeed stands out from the pack of other fitness models, so much so that many do not call it a gym or program—they actually call it a cult.

SUMMARIZING THE DEFINITION:

- X-Company is a very popular exercise routine that is done across the globe.

- More than seven thousand gyms (boxes) are affiliate members.

- X-Company is a business: each affiliate member gym must pay a yearly fee, along with its trainers, who must pay a certification fee in order to train.

- X-Company has a ten-year partnership with Reebok® (owned by Adidas). Reebok® provides financial backing for X-Company Games, and X-Company has its own line of apparel.

- X-Company is growing, branching away from young, healthy, and fit— it is now marketing to nearly everyone.

Chapter 2: The Cult

"It can kill you," he said.
"I've always been completely honest about that."

— Greg Glassman, founder of X-Company, in an interview with the New York Times.

Food is an essential building block for our body. Food is more than energy—it is life, nutrients, and a social experience. Exercise can also be seen in similar abstract perspectives. Exercise can make the old feel young, bring life to feeble muscles, and unite a group of people to sweat together for success. You likely have a concept of what defines your food and exercise from your own perspective. Your definition of food comes from your culture, your family, and your environment. Exercise behaviors are shaped in a similar way. The diet and exercise culture differs among those in X-Company—let's look at how they are different.

The Caveman

In the past century no other culture in the world has trended upon so many diet fads as the Western world. Most diets orient themselves around a food group, the timing of food, or ratio of certain foods to others. The reasoning for these diets was mostly rooted in mysticism, trends, or culture. In the last sixty years it has become apparent that diets have becoming a booming business.

X-Company has built a culture of what foods to eat within their facilities. To call it caveman-like is fairly accurate because the selection of foods is rudimentary, as is the preparation of the meals. The X-Company website makes it clear that a diet should be simple. It outlines this breakdown of nutrients:

Food Group	Percent of Daily Total Calories
Lean and Varied Protein	30 percent
Monounsaturated Fats	30 percent
Low-Glycemic Carbohydrates	40 percent

Calories are determined based on 0.7 to 1.0 grams of protein per pound of lean body mass, depending on your activity level. The 0.7-gram level is for moderate exercise, while the 1.0-gram level is for intense exercise.

The diet is simple and clear until you reach the last row regarding how to determine your total caloric intake. The total calorie determination is biased toward an athlete's dietary prescription and may not be appropriate for individuals with kidney issues or the general population. The X-Company website goes further in saying, "In plain language, base your diet on garden vegetables, especially greens, lean meats, nuts and seeds, little starch, and no sugar. That's about as simple as we can get." X-Company gives further specifics on how food should be a "living" organism and how to focus your shopping on the peripherals of a store (most stores stock perishable foods on the perimeter of the store). These are great, generalized recommendations. Moreover, the website states that you should avoid eating large number of calories, a concept called caloric restriction.

I am intimately familiar with the benefits of caloric restriction. Having co-authored one undergraduate and one graduate-level research study on the benefits of longevity and caloric restriction, I have seen and measured the merits of eating less. X-Company seems to have some solid dietary recommendations. But what is the foundation for this diet?

X-Company has adopted the "Paleolithic" diet, also known as "Paleo," as its official diet of choice. The concept of this diet is that our bodies have not evolved quickly enough to adapt to the modernization of the food industry. In other words, your body cannot properly process the foods you are eating because it has had too little of time to change. As such, the Paleo diet purports that the majority of foods you should eat are those that can be either hunted or gathered.

But what is the science supporting this conjecture? Currently there are no peer-reviewed, scientific publications testing the Paleo diet's rationale. There has been one study examining the effects of a Paleo diet on blood cholesterol values. This study showed "deleterious changes in blood lipids for healthy subjects" (Eric Trexler. "Paleolithic Diet is associated with unfavorable changes to blood lipids in healthy subjects." [2013]. http://hdl.handle.net/1811/54660). These findings showed that a Paleo diet can increase the "bad" cholesterol (LDL), and increase the overall total cholesterol in healthy subjects. As cholesterol and LDL values trend higher, a person is at greater risk of developing a heart attack or stroke.

It should be noted that this study was conducted after ten weeks of eating a Paleo diet while performing X-Company. The author did find that the subjects had a better fitness status and body-fat percentage at the end of the ten weeks; however, these improvements may not outweigh the rising cholesterol levels over time, especially when the risk for cardiovascular heart disease increases with higher LDL levels. A longer and larger study is needed to test whether the higher blood values have a significant impact on health, despite the lower body fat and improved fitness level.

Myriad books, blogs, and websites are dedicated to the Paleo diet. It appears that everyone is an expert and has found the silver bullet to ending chronic diseases in this country — this cure-all (there's that word again) being the Paleo diet. However, scientists and licensed dieticians alike are not convinced that the Paleo diet is the be-all and end-all diet.

Major anecdotal concerns exist with the Paleo diet. One of these is the heavy emphasis on animal-based proteins. A person on the Paleo diet may think like this: well, if a caveman would have eaten this food, so should I. The logic may go further: instead of eating a bagel, which is processed food, I will eat this entire package of bacon — after all, it is animal protein that a caveman would eat. This may seem like good logic until you realize that a person has substituted a large portion of his or her varied diet of vegetables, fruits, nuts, and grains with a single category of meat, eggs, and dairy. The overzealousness and promotion of meat consumption smell a lot like another diet plan that was misunderstood in the not-too-distant past: the Atkins diet.

The number of people on the Paleo diet who overconsume meat has not been measured or published in the literature. As such, it is hard to tell if this concern happens in a high enough number of Paleo dieters to warrant a change in their recommendations. However, it is interesting to see the measured increases in the blood cholesterol levels of twenty-three males and twenty females in the ten week study referenced above. Could this be a result of overeating meat? Further research is needed to establish any cause and effect.

The concept of avoiding certain foods in a diet has great merit. A person on a strict Paleo diet will embrace vegetables, nuts, and lean meats, while shunning processed foods, high-glycemic carbohydrates, and heavy saturated fats. These are fabulous guidelines, but only when implemented correctly. More evidence is emerging on the avoidance of certain foods containing gluten, dairy (cow's milk), and renin. Gluten can cause inflammatory responses and promote central obesity (Ana Izcue, Janine L. Coombes, and Fiona Powrie. "Regulatory T cells suppress systemic and mucosal immune activation to control intestinal inflammation." Immunological Reviews 212.1 [2006]: 256–271). Moreover, a gluten-free diet has been shown to increase bone density in patients with osteoporosis (Valentina Passananti et al. "Bone mass in women with celiac disease: Role of exercise and gluten-free diet." Digestive and Liver Disease 44.5 [2012]: 379–383). In addition, dairy from cows has been shown to promote gut problems (Michael I. Goran, and T. L. Alderete. "Targeting adipose tissue inflammation to treat the underlying basis of the metabolic complications of obesity." [2012]: 49–60) and myriad other issues such as type 1 diabetes, autism, heart disease, and acne. The website www.greenmedinfo.com/toxic-ingredient/cow-milk lists several major peer-reviewed scientific publications on dairy and its negative consequences.

It could be true that our bodies were not ready or designed by God to process modern-day dairy and gluten. Perhaps the evolution of the food industry has altered the most basic and fundamental foods to a point where our bodies nearly reject the food they were designed to digest. Or perhaps humans were never meant to consume these foods at all. Research and open-minded clinicians will guide us to the best practices for each individual.

The X-Company website encourages participants to seriously examine the Paleolithic diet because "The Caveman model is perfectly consistent with the X-Company prescription." What is the best process of examining this diet? The X-Company website asks participants to pull websites from Google to read the best "compelling and extensive" findings. The lack of scientific publications focusing on Paleo should be obvious to the objective and logical reader. Google may be a good resource; however, it is not the foundation for solid dietary-based recommendations for athletes, let alone people with medical issues. We will observe X-Company exercisers researching items on their own in the subsection ahead, as they attempt to "heal" their own physical injuries. The continual theme of turning away from science and the peer-reviewed publications and guidelines is ever-present within the X-Company community. Regardless of X-Company's research strategy, however, it does appear that the Paleo diet may be on to some solid recommendations.

It begs the question as to why X-Company has turned away from the more substantiated Mediterranean diet, which has scientific merit within the peer-reviewed literature and mirrors many of the principles of the Paleo diet. A five-year study of nearly eight thousand people found that a Mediterranean diet can cut a person's heart disease risk by 30 percent (Ramon Estruch et al. "Effects of a Mediterranean-style diet on cardiovascular risk factors: A randomized trial." Annals of Internal Medicine 145.1 [2006]: 1–11). The Mediterranean diet also embraces common themes of minimizing gluten and dairy, both positive factors. The data is still out on the Paleo diet's benefits—apparently X-Company wants to force the Paleo on its constituents. As newbie X-Company exercisers often discover, the model of forcefulness can be found in many of the "boxes" in several ways.

You Big Pussy

X-Company involves group exercise, which offers both positive and negative components. The positive components can include peer-to-peer competition and encouragement, better profit margins for the box, and a sense of "unity." The negative aspects may be directly related to those positive aspects of X-Company's take on group exercise.

I interviewed several friends who trialed the X-Company experience. Some reported that the training staff and fellow X-Company exercisers were overly competitive, pushy, and forceful at times. They said they were pushed beyond their physiological levels and comfort zones through peer pressure and ostracizing. One box utilized a large public board that allowed participants to tout their heaviest Olympic lifts. My friend felt that the board either served as public humiliation if you were not lifting heavy weight or as sheer bragging when the weight lifted was extreme.

The underlying tones of this forceful and manipulative mantra can be seen on several affiliate X-Company gym's websites. Larry Palazzolo wrote an article titled, "Ten Tips for the Success of an X-Company Newbie." The article begins by describing the odd scene that you will likely encounter in a X-Company box"

> You might see a bunch of half-naked hard bodies showing off their ink and abs, ripping out butterfly kip after butterfly kip. You might ask yourself, "Is that person having a seizure or doing pull-ups? What's with all the Chuck Taylors? Do they get a group rate? What's with the guy in the corner wearing only sweatpants, shirt off, all tatted up and muttering to himself? Is he on a work release program?"

X-Company may not offer the welcoming environment you are looking for, at least according to Palazzolo's article. His article continues by explaining in Tip 1 how individual X-Company exercisers should only compare their performance to only themselves. A new exerciser should "go at their own pace" and "let the intensity find you." These seem like reasonable recommendations for experienced lifters and exercisers. But these are newbies; how do they know when and where to begin, let alone how to properly "dose" their exercise? Later in the book we will discuss how exercise should be properly prescribed based on national guidelines.

Rule 2 outlines how one should learn to "scale," which is the X-Company term for increasing or decreasing the intensity of an exercise. Larry's recommendations for scaling are to "know your own body and its limits" and that "there's no substitute for common sense." How would anyone know their limits if they have not been assessed or educated on their specific limits? Large majorities of people who begin to exercise stop the exercise journey because of exercising too much at first—soreness or an injury deters them from becoming lifelong exercisers.

I challenge you to think about the last time you began an exercise program or a new exercise routine. How comfortable were you in knowing your limits? Did you seek the guidance of a certified personal trainer or physical therapist to gain better parameters on your intensity? These would be reasonable, prudent, and commonsense approaches to exercising for a newbie. Perhaps Larry and most of the X-Company community have left their common sense in the corner with the drooling meathead he described in his article.

Just like not all gyms are the same, not all X-Company boxes are the same. In my X-Company experience in South Florida, the group that was exercising performed their lifts and moves in relative silence, with the exception of the obvious panting and occasional grunting. I did not hear people cheering each other, but I did see the coach provide some motivational cues to individuals who were struggling. I did not see drooling tattooed men, but I saw young kids, beautiful women, and overly developed suave men. I am sure the business owners curtail their boxes to meet the needs of the surrounding population—in the box I tried, most were middle-class to upper-middle-class, educated, white people. Several donned university sweatshirts and jumped into their sports cars or luxury sport utility vehicles after their workout—this may be very different from your box in downtown Detroit or Los Angeles.

Haters and the People of X-Company

Several websites, blogs, and forums delineate the many reasons why people hate X-Company (www.ihatecrossfit, http://forum.bodybuilding.com/showthread.php? t=148982113&page=1, http://board.crossfit.com/showthread.php?t=77977). A top reason people steer clear of a box is the atmosphere. Several claim that having a group of people cheering you on while you sweat, puke, or pass out is not appealing. Furthermore, the competitive nature, not just during the exercise portion, can be seen through idolatry of shoes, socks, and outfits. While this latter notion can be seen in most sports or organized activities, an attitude called "holier-than-thou" can be pervasive among many X-Company exercisers. A person with the holier-than-thou attitude believes that all non-X-Company exercisers are below them. It is this self-righteous attitude that can quickly turn away newbies and leave many feeling unwelcomed.

Examining the demographics of the 2010 X-Company Games shows the average male and female ages were twenty-eight and twenty-nine years old, respectively. As cited in many online sources, people feel the atmosphere in the box is uplifting and supporting—some may call it pushy. Regardless, there is constant, immediate external feedback. Moreover, the supporters and "success stories" of X-Company cite the amazingly quick results from the routine, especially compared to traditional exercise. The atmosphere of constant positive reinforcement along with the allure of fast results from exercise seems to align with the values of people born in the Generation X (1980–1992). Generation X has had a high exposure to technology with instantaneous results. These individuals have a tendency to want things now, with continual pats on the back (whether good or bad form is in place)—it is a generation that may be easily susceptible to what some call a cult.

The X-Company atmosphere may work for some individuals looking for an over supportive group of self-righteous individuals; of course, these behaviors may fluctuate from box to box. Research supports that effective group exercise includes positive reinforcement and modeling; however, I think X-Company's bad apples (as described on X-Company's forums) tend to perpetuate the concept that the X-Company population is in fact a cult. They worship their trinity of food, exercise, and rest. They congregate in one location for a set purpose. And they are willing to look down on you, the non-X-Company exercisers, as if you were an atheist lost in the middle of a crusade. The quick results and constant positive reinforcement are certainly alluring if you are among the younger generation. However, the question must be asked: at what physical cost?

Circular Injury Management

"It can kill you," he said. "I've always been completely honest about that."
—Greg Glassman, in an interview with the New York Times

If X-Company does not kill you, you may find yourself injured at some point. Again, with no professional organizational structure, X-Company has not gleaned longitudinal data to report injuries or cite prevalence of conditions following X-Company in the short or long term. Any exerciser will tell you that he or she has had some injury at some point in training—X-Company exercisers, especially. Where did the X-Company exercisers go for treatment of their injuries? They reported back to the X-Company box.

Circular injury management is a common practice among X-Company exercisers. The concept of circular injury management is simple: you train, you get injured, you return for more training in hope of alleviating your symptoms. No physician, no medications, just the trinity: food, rest, and exercise.

Injury management can be in the form of stretching or more lifts and punishing exercises. It should be noted, after referencing the X-Company Level 1 Trainers' Guidebook, that X-Company trainers have not been trained like physical therapists. A physical therapist has the education and training to provide the most skilled rehabilitation following an injury. We will discuss educational competencies in a later chapter.

Regardless, the staff cannot, legally speaking, direct physical therapy services. Moreover, the staff has not been educated to assess injuries or provide proper rehabilitation-level care. Therefore, if you are X-Company exercisers with an injury, you can expect to remain with the pack and be guided by those who think they know what they are doing. Most of the guidance from X-Company staff comes from what they have seen in other participants' injury experiences and from what they themselves have had to recover from.

Dr. Hashish, a physical therapist, wrote about a common saying within X-Company boxes: "death by…" as in "death by push-ups." Dr. Hashish said this term is
> …an obvious exaggeration that in X-Company terminology means to add a single repetition each successive minute until failure. However, the term, and this method of exercise, symbolizes the X-Company mantra of forging elite fitness, seemingly by pushing yourself past your preconceived limit. (http://www.huffingtonpost.com/ rami-hashish/crossfit-debate_b_3181435.html)

Dr. Hashish makes an affirmation that X-Company should not be the exercise of choice due to the high likelihood of injury and the lack of supporting research.

A good friend of mine is an X-Company exerciser. He has training in sports medicine and is an orthopedic physician's assistant. He spent years in the operating room and orthopedic clinics treating patients with common muscle pulls, fractures, and arthritis. Despite his background and education he has chosen X-Company as his means of exercise. He remarks that it is the best workout he has had. The only issues he cannot remedy are his continual muscle pulls in his calf. He sought my attention to help remedy his dysfunction.

I asked him several questions including what would cause his pain, when it first happened, how he was exercising, and what he had done to treat it — very common questions during a physical therapist's examination. Sprinting caused his pain and also made it reoccur. He had continued his X-Company routine, but his coach guided him to reduce his intensity, perform copious stretches of that muscle, and aggressively massage his calf. His own orthopedic knowledge helped guide him to some degree; however, despite his knowledge and coach's tips, his calf continued to cause him pain while sprinting. Prior to meeting me, he had never sought the care of a physician or physical therapist.

The issue he had was a recurring muscle strain due to aggressive forces during sprinting. As the muscle would heal, he would begin training and stretching it aggressively too soon. As a result, he would retear the muscle, and he would be back at square one again (if not worse). The interesting thing I noted about his treatment regimen (exercise) was that it did not include any calf-specific muscle training. He loaded the calf forcefully only during large, gross movements like running and jumping. He spent no time on specific calf muscle training like calf raises—more will be discussed later on the flawed training methods of X-Company. Suffice it to say my friend was caught in circular injury management.

Later in the book you will read about a gentleman named John who unfortunately suffered a major medical issue after doing X-Company. Prior to John seeking medical care, he spoke with his X-Company trainer. John recalled, "I sent her a text message after I couldn't straighten my arms because of pain and stiffness. Her response was that it was soreness and that I should return to the box for another workout." It is obvious that the X-Company facility was either trying to "manage" his condition or was simply not well educated in his exercise-induced condition. What John needed was not another workout—he needed a hospital. Injuries during exercise come in many forms. Orthopedic injuries such as my friend's muscle strain are the most common. Injuries to the nerves, heart, and even pelvic floor can occur, and often these even more serious injuries warrant further medical follow-up.

A good example of an injury to the pelvic floor is stress urinary incontinence. Stress urinary incontinence can be a common dysfunction following pregnancy (David H. Thom and Guri Rortveit. "Prevalence of postpartum urinary incontinence: a systematic review." Acta Obstetricia et Gynecologica Scandinavica 89.12 [2010]: 1511–1522); however, it can also occur in people who have not borne children. Stress urinary incontinence is when a person cannot maintain tone in the pelvic floor muscles to appropriately restrict the flow of urine during a stressful movement (e.g., lifting heavy weights, coughing, or standing). The incontinence is often embarrassing and can lead to other complications if not properly addressed. According to the X-Company culture, stress urinary incontinence is acceptable, funny, and a "normal" process.

Do you pee during your workouts? According to several female X-Company participants in a YouTube video, they often urinate during their workouts due to the extreme stress of lifting (http://www.youtube.com/watch?v=UKzq1upNIgU). In the video many of the ladies laugh, embracing the fact and commenting on it as if it were a medal they had earned. At the time of writing this book, more than 320,000 people had viewed this video—you too can view it by searching "do you pee during workouts" on the X-Company channel of YouTube (or by using the link provided above).

There has been a strong response against the video from several individuals and organizations. A physical therapist wrote a scathing article about X-Company and cited the "peeing" video (http://www.huffingtonpost.com/eric-robertson/crossfit-rhabdomyolysis_b_3977598.html).

His bottom-line summary: urinating while you lift is not a normal phenomenon. The American Physical Therapy Association (APTA) and the Australian Physiotherapy Association (APA) both created separate but direct responses to the X-Company YouTube video (http://www.moveforwardpt.com/Radio/Detail.aspx?cid=ae96ec2e-b894-4bae-a8e2-2c504a5f0bb4 and http://www.physiotherapy.asn.au/APAWCM/The_APA/news/June_2013/crossfit_Games_sends_disturbing_message.aspx). The APTA and APA make it clear that urinating during lifting is not a normal condition. Furthermore, they make the clear argument for proper diagnosis, treatment, and prevention. The best specialist to see for this issue is a women's health physical therapist. These physical therapists train and specialize in women's health, which encompasses pelvic floor reeducation, modalities to relax or stimulate muscles, and education for improving your condition. You can search for these professionals at the American Board of Physical Therapy Specialties (ABPTS) at www.abpts.org.

X-Company's approach to modifying its participants' thinking by acceptance of a bodily dysfunction such as stress urinary incontinence demonstrates how a culture can alter the truth to maintain its numbers and image. Whether you are banging on your chest like a caveman, screaming at your buddy lifting more weight than his body can ever handle, or peeing on the floor while performing an Olympic lift, you just learned that the cult of X-Company has you right where it wants you—in their wallet.

IN SUMMARY:

- X-Company endorses the Paleo diet, which focuses on nonprocessed, basic foods.

- The Paleo diet has merit, although its effects have not been as well proven as a somewhat similar diet, the Mediterranean diet. The Mediterranean diet is the subject of several well-researched articles and the backing of many cardiologists. Choose the Mediterranean diet over the Paleo diet.

- X-Company exercisers have a unique culture, which can seem overbearing to some. The constant positive reinforcement and push to do more exercise is ever-present—this often appeals to the younger generations.

- X-Company embraces a "holier-than-thou" attitude.

- The X-Company culture is biased to their cultural norm to such a degree that even urinating on the floor while lifting is acceptable.

- Urinating while lifting is called stress urinary incontinence. It is not a normal response to exercise and warrants further medical treatment, particularly by a woman's health physical therapist. Seek medical advice if you become injured during or after X-Company.

Chapter 3: The Design, the Dollar, and the Diploma?

"X-Company's gross revenue approached roughly $20 million for 2012."

"X-Company Inc. does not accredit, inspect, or measure the success of affiliate gyms. As such, the only requirement for a box to begin and continue to educate new trainers every year is money."

Program Design

You may not know the name Lee-Ann Ellison, but you may have seen her picture. She made national news when she posted her pictures on Facebook performing Olympic lifts and kettlebell swings (http://well.blogs.nytimes.com/2013/09/24/pregnant-weight-lifter-stirs-debate/?_r=0). These moves involve raising a heavy barbell over her head and swinging a large weighted ball with handle well over her head repeatedly. She was performing these exercises as part of her commitment to the cult of X-Company. You might ask what the issue was—she is exercising like so many Americans fail to do, right? Well, Lee-Ann was doing these dangerous and skilled movements while eight months pregnant.

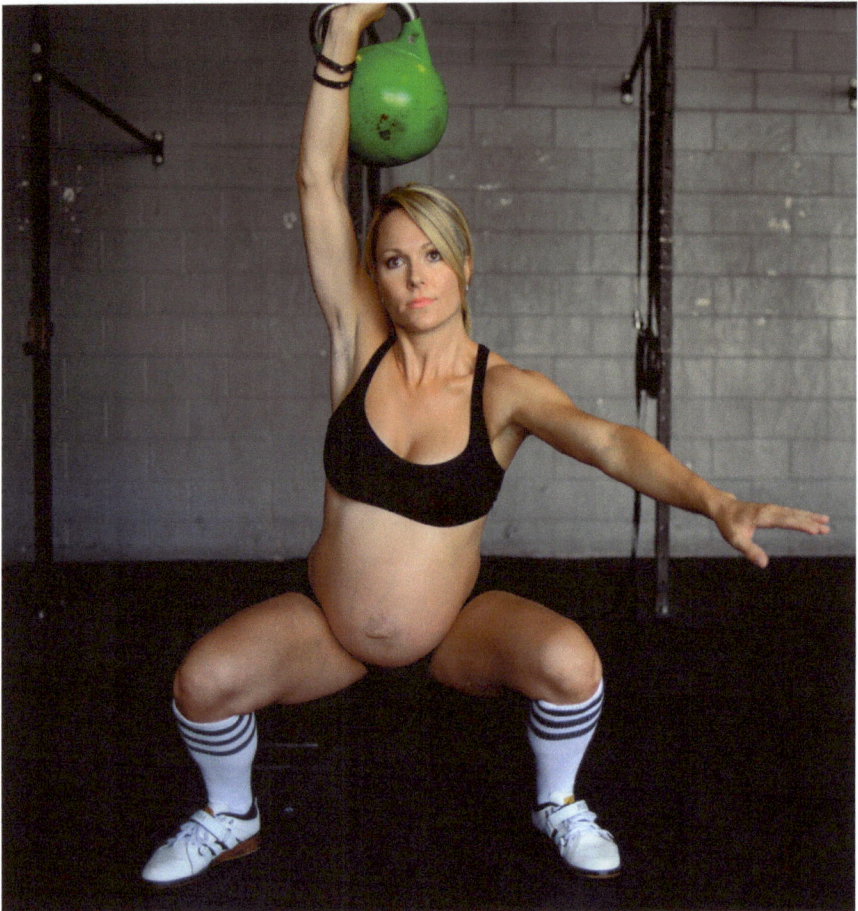

Lee-Ann Ellison performs an overhead kettlebell move.

(permission to use by Wenn Inc.)

The pictures of Lee-Ann stirred much debate, comments, and press. Several other pregnant X-Company exercisers came forward to speak about how X-Company had helped them stay fit and healthy while pregnant. Meanwhile, other pregnant women spoke about how they chose an alternative exercise path, which included following national exercise guidelines for pregnant women. Members of this latter group posted to express shock and even criticism.

Kudos to the women of X-Company for bringing the importance of exercise during pregnancy to the mainstream media via viral means. The press certainly covered the mixed emotions on the topic and brought in several "specialists" to weigh in with their opinions. For instance, the New York Times quoted Dr. Daniel Roshan, an assistant professor at New York University Medical School and a maternal fetal medicine specialist, saying "pregnant women should be careful not to push their heart rates above 140 beats per minute or raise their body temperatures above 100 degrees Fahrenheit. The goal is to avoid exercising to exhaustion."

Dr. Roshan remarked that heavy lifting should be discouraged during pregnancy, as it can stimulate early delivery. He further commented that it was obvious that Lee-Ann was in excellent shape and had been lifting in this style for some time. I question

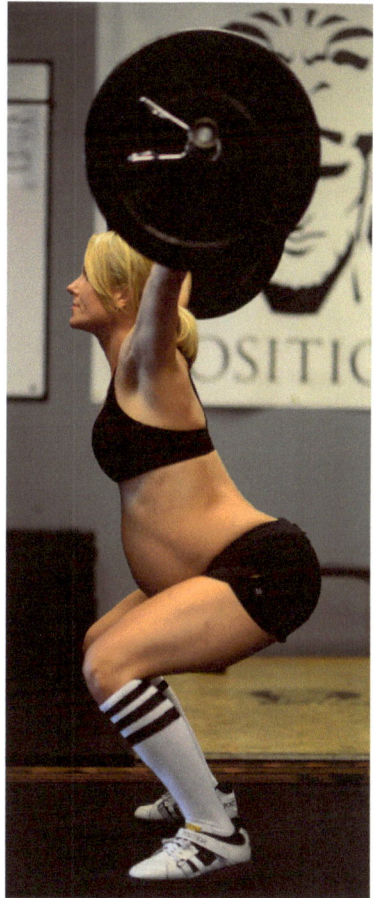

Lee-Ann in the snatch
(permission to use by Wenn Inc.)

how Dr. Roshan could determine a woman's fitness status or expertise in lifts based on still photos alone. These are exercise movements, not holding poses with weights. Furthermore, Dr. Roshan, a well-published assistant professor and medical doctor, holds a background in primarily in obstetrics and gynecology, not exercise. Based on his curriculum vitae, he holds no credentialing in exercise performance and movement assessment.

In spite of these comments, Dr. Roshan does make an argument based on scientific evidence that women nurses who work twelve-hour shifts are more likely to give birth to earlier and lighter babies than nurses who work only eight-hour shifts. The argument here is that the bodies of the nurses who work longer shifts shunt important nutrients from the baby to the mother's body. The notion of mild to moderate exertion and exercise makes sense and is supported by Dr. Roshan, and more importantly, by national guidelines.

So who failed in providing Lee-Ann and others with these appropriate guidelines to safeguard themselves and their children?

The answer is simple: the X-Company trainers. The role of a certified personal trainer is assessment, development, prescription, and progression of exercise, while maintaining safety standards. At the current time, no evidenced-based articles support the notion of high-intensity exercise, let alone "X-Company-style" exercise, as safe for pregnant women. As such, it is the duty of the X-Company trainer to err on the side of caution. Physical therapists often subscribe to the Hippocratic Oath, part of which is "never do harm." X-Company trainers have no such oath.

Where is the criticism of the trainers in the New York Times article? Dr. Roshan cites national guidelines on maintaining a heart rate below 140 beats per minute; however, the article does not even touch on one of the most important steps before exercise, the pre-exercise screening and assessment.

Pre-exercise Screening

X-Company has been notorious for allowing individuals of all shape, size, and fitness statuses to show up at their boxes and start throwing weights around—sometimes for free. The allure of this amazing deal is appealing: free exercise is great, right? The issue is that your free session likely lacks the necessary pre-exercise screening. Beyond freebies, anecdotal evidence shows that X-Company boxes are guilty of not performing pre-exercise screenings or assessments for many of their clients. Consider this akin to your physician writing you a prescription for a powerful drug without examining you or your lab results. Wouldn't you hold this physician accountable when your health fails?

Pre-exercise screening and assessment are very important for preventing injury, establishing objective goals, and prescribing exercise. The American College of Sports Medicine (ACSM) has been a leader in establishing the safe and effective way to assess and screen clients before exercise. In fact, ACSM has entire texts, which are updated frequently, dedicated to assessment and pre-exercise screening.

During the screening process with an exercise specialist, a person identifies active signs or symptoms suggestive of disease. These can include shortness of breath, swelling of the ankles, or heart palpitations—the list is long but reasonable enough to identify those with active diseases that may warrant further medical testing by a physician. A screening process can include a simple preparticipation questionnaire or PAR-Q for short, which is best used for those who are about to engage in moderate physical activity. PAR-Qs are most commonly used incorrectly by X-Company facilities. The questionnaire should only be used for moderate physical activity—X-Company is high-intensity physical activity. Perform a search online for "X-Company and PAR-Q" and you will see how prevalent this document has become in X-Company facilities. In short, more robust questionnaires and an interview processes should be used prior to exercising with a trainer, especially if the exercise is at high intensities.

Ideally, what is fostered by the ACSM, the National Strength and Conditioning Association (NSCA), and the American Physical Therapy Association (APTA), is the use of a health history questionnaire coupled with a client interview. A health history questionnaire details a person's prior medical issues, current medical issues, medications, as well as other factors such as substance abuse, social factors, and health/performance goals. Simply listing these items is not sufficient—clarification is often needed and is essential for proper assessment and screening.

After the interview and health history questionnaire is complete, a personal trainer should then be able to classify you based on your risk for a cardiovascular event. In a process known as risk stratification, the personal trainer or exercise specialist will classify you as low, moderate, or high risk for having a cardiac event based on whether you have active signs of disease and the number of risk factors you have for heart disease. The latter include high cholesterol, high blood pressure, and age.

> ## THE CLASSIFICATION SYSTEM HAS A PURPOSE:
>
> 1. It limits the person's exercise intensity if he or she is at high risk.
>
> 2. It can signal to the exercise specialist that further monitoring is needed during exercise (e.g., heart rate monitoring, watching oxygen levels, blood pressure checks).
>
> 3. It requires a physician to be present during exercise (in certain states and situations) if the person is at high risk.

Anecdotal evidence suggests that no X-Company facilities perform this kind of risk stratification, and a health history questionnaire is not a standard part of its operating procedures. Scouring X-Company's online "journal," there is no evidence of articles supporting the use of this safety system for preventing sudden cardiac arrest. During my X-Company "assessment," which included basically four days of varying exercises, I was never questioned by my trainer on my medical issues. I occasionally mentioned some of my prior injuries during several movements in hopes this would prime his curiosity, but my mentioning of injuries spurred very little other than "Stop if it hurts."

Prior to exercising, I signed my initials in roughly five spots on a waiver stating, "I am healthy" or "I have seen a physician." Initialing these statements do not benefit or protect the client—in most cases it also does not completely waive a company's liability. The bottom line: X-Company provides poor pre-exercise screening for it participants, which places its members at risk and is a disservice to those who need further medical help.

The exercise and rehabilitation fields have gone to lengths to establish such algorithms and systems to keep people safe to make itself more credible to the community. In not properly screening and taking a history of its clients, X-Company undermines the progress made in the professions of exercise.

One may argue that many of the "big-box" centers in the fitness industry mimic what X-Company does for pre-exercise screening. I have spoken with other trainers, students, and colleagues who have worked at these large facilities that are focused on volume of exercisers. It appears that many trainers, although educated in health screening/stratification techniques, often do not perform them. They often cite laziness, difficulty, or questions about the need for such questionnaires and screenings. While I have no objective data on the prevalence of such risky behavior, I will argue that the exercise done in the large gym is significantly less intense than exercise done in an X-Company box. I think even an X-Company exercisers would agree with my last statement. As such, you may not be screened in either the X-Company box or big gym, but you may be more likely to have sudden cardiac arrest in the X-Company box— simply due to the high intensity of the exercise.

Beyond the risk stratification and health history, the initial assessment provides a framework for a personal trainer to establish objective goals. These goals should be meaningful and easily measured, such as a person's percentage of body fat, lower- and upper-body strength, and blood pressure. From these measures an exercise prescription can be made that will establish a program for that specific individual's needs. Furthermore, the trainer and client can set reasonable goals to work toward in that exercise program—a commonsense approach. The ACSM has an entire text on guidelines for exercise testing and prescription. In the event the argument is made that these measures are not sport or athletic appropriate, look toward NSCA as it has guidelines for testing athletes. X-Company's excuse that the fitness and sport world does not provide reasonable, clear, and practical guidelines for more intense exercise is ridiculously unfounded.

Group Exercise

"The trainer handed me a pink piece of chalk and told me to write my name and weight lifted on the chalkboard. I refused. The trainer then told me to continue doing push-ups, pull-ups, and squats. I was spent—he pushed me to keep going. I ran for the bathroom in an excuse to catch my breath and rest my body. I returned and the trainer asked me to keep going…I told him to go fuck himself and I left."

Jim, a friend and caregiver to a patient of mine, gave me this excerpt after an in-home PT session with his step-dad. Jim had recently attended an X-Company program in our town in order to lose some weight. Jim is a believer in alternative medicine, safe supplementation, and exercise; however, he had never seen something as ridiculous or dangerous as X-Company.

Jim remarked, "It's a bunch of people of grunting, throwing weights around, swinging kettlebells in the air—a group session of intense exercise."

Jim identified one of the biggest flaws with the programming of X-Company: it's a group exercise approach. Scientific journals have demonstrated the benefits of inpatient group physical therapy exercise, group wellness classes for seniors, and group cardio sessions for those looking to lose weight. These programs have been safely developed under the guidelines of large, national organization such as the ACSM or the American Council of Exercise (ACE). Furthermore, these programs have further been tested through longitudinal trials and copious case series examining safety. After publications, and usually at the yearly national conferences, these programs are further refined and shaped into cohesive, safe, and effective exercise delivery systems. X-Company, at this time, has done none of these steps to ensure the safety of its programming. It is simple: bring your money, sign on the dotted line, and start throwing weights around in a group setting. You might ask, what's the issue with this?

The intensity of the movements done in X-Company warrants very close monitoring of its participants. Consider the training for a football player, something that X-Company exercisers often cite as a similar exercise programming to that of X-Company (which it is not). The professional football player in the National Football League has been screened by the sports medicine team. The sports medicine team includes athletic trainers, orthopedist, general medical doctors, and strength and conditioning specialists. These experts examine the athletes for injuries, illnesses, weaknesses, and anything that can be prevented or treated. All of this is done before practice or team lifts (e.g., high-intensity group exercise). None of these are currently required to participate in X-Company. Therefore, the similarity of other safe and effective group exercise programs, such as those done by professional athletes and military personnel, to X-Company is unfounded. Another key difference between professional football players and X-Company exercisers: the football players are training toward a goal, whereas the X-Company exerciser is merely exercising.

In other settings where group exercise has proven to be effective, such as inpatient rehabilitation and outpatient cardiac rehabilitation, licensed health-care providers examine the participants of group exercise sessions. Moreover, trained, certified, and educated exercise specialists monitor the participants continually, utilizing technology such as blood pressure cuffs, heart rate monitors, and oxygen sensors.

In the fitness or wellness setting, a certified group fitness instructor can safely lead a group class without extensive pre-exercise screening. The group fitness instructor achieves this by:

1. making it clear that the exercise is voluntary;

2. forewarning those with medical conditions or movement issues that they refrain from certain movements or the class altogether;

3. providing exercise modifications for those struggling to keep form; and

4. keeping the exercise intensity at a safe level for all who participate.

Could X-Company adapt its ways to meet these? Possibly, but it may be challenging due to X-Company's consistent high-intensity group exercise for everyone. Understand that gyms, fitness facilities, and wellness centers often provide tiered class systems for their exercisers. This allows novice exercisers a way to progress and not get injured early in their journey to better health and fitness.

Exercise modification, another tool used by exercise specialists to promote creativity and a well-balanced training approach, is often not embraced in the X-Company programming. In one-on-one sessions and group sessions, exercise specialists sometimes must modify an exercise because of poor form. During my X-Company "trial," I noticed several participants struggling with heavy weights, having poor form, and having no coach cuing them. X-Company purportedly prides itself on proper form. I question how this can be achieved in a group setting when there are more participants, exercising at extreme intensities, than trainers. Moreover, X-Company's movements are complex—many muscles and joints are coordinating all at once. X-Company has too many extreme movements and too many participants with not enough well-trained eyes. X-Company's approach is to not modify the program but to reinforce that this is the program and you *will* be sticking to it!

The programming of X-Company does not permit safe, individualized exercise for all participants with varied health histories and fitness statuses. Group exercise has proven to be efficacious in other settings where pre-exercise screening is in place, rigorous monitoring can be done, and trained professionals can intervene when appropriate. It is obvious that such intense exercise requires further pre-exercise testing and screening, along with appropriate monitoring of all parties at increased risk. Why would X-Company use this format of training? The programming has permitted X-Company to grow rapidly and become extremely profitable. The group exercise concept allows for minimal staff, maximizes the flow of clients, and ensures profitability. Let's look at X-Company as not just an exercise routine but as a *company*.

The Company

"Today, X-Company, the company, provides accredited training seminars throughout the world" (http://www.crossfit.com/cf-info/certs.shtml). After reading this sentence, the true definition of X-Company should be apparent: it is a company with a global mission. X-Company currently licenses the name "X-Company." A gym that would like to offer X-Company-style training or establish a business name that incorporates the word "X-Company" must pay X-Company Inc. an annual fee of $3,000. X-Company Inc. calls this an "affiliation."

To be an affiliate gym, a business owner must complete an application process. The application includes an essay of why the applicant wants to open a gym. Another prerequisite is that the applicant be a certified X-Company Level 1 Instructor. The certificate involves a weekend course with an instructor where an instructor reviews the X-Company movements, provides technique feedback for the attendees on their own movements, and educates on how to "scale." Scaling means to make an exercise more or less intense (in the exercise science world, we call this prescribe or "dose"). The cost for this weekend course is $1,000—a $250 deposit is required to even register, with payments accepted up until the time the course is offered. X-Company Inc. does not accredit, inspect, or measure the success of these affiliate gyms. As such, the only requirement for a box to begin and continue to educate new trainers every year is money.

Other courses and continuing education regarding X-Company will be discussed in further detail later. However, it is clear that X-Company Inc. has done a fabulous job utilizing its affiliate facilities to scale (pun intended) its business model. The company utilizes these affiliates to teach its courses and maintain a consistent online presence: the same registration system, an identical payment processing system, and duplicated copy and images.

Examining these numbers conservatively, we find that the recurring revenue is robust. The rate of growth of X-Company gyms has been cited by some as nearly doubling every few years (Huntley, CrossFit Forums). Given this assumption and the above rates, let's do some quick math:

ESTIMATED REVENUE FOR X-COMPANY IN ONE YEAR BASED ON AFFILIATE FEES IN 2013

Item	Cost to Affiliate	Number of Facilities Paying	Total
Startup Costs for New Gyms Each Year	$4,000	300	$1.2 million
Renewing Gym Affiliate Fees	$3,000	6,100 (globally)	$18.3 million
			$19.5 million gross revenue each year

These numbers do not include revenue from other intermediate and advanced certifications that X-Company offers. Tim Huntley of My Athletic Life has estimated that X-Company's gross revenue approached roughly $20 million for 2012 (http://myathleticlife.com/2012/02/crossfit-worth-500-million/). Even more, Tim conjectures X-Company's total expenses to be at or below 50 percent of gross revenue—this equates to nearly $10 million in profits for 2012!

X-Company worked a deal with Reebok® to present the X-Company Games after establishing a partnership in 2010 (http://www.bloomberg.com/news/2013-05-29/adidas-to-make-crossfit-delta-logo-symbol-for-reebok-fitness.html). The purpose of these games is to find "the fittest person in the world." The cable channel ESPN3 is where X-Company exercisers and fans can watch these games, which are oriented around world rankings based on weight lifted and time to complete groupings of exercises. The television exposure has certainly bolstered, if not expanded, the brand of X-Company.

Also included in the ten-year Reebok®–X-Company partnership is X-Company's own line of apparel that that began selling in fall of 2011. An intriguing piece of apparel that has sold well is a "specialized" X-Company shoe. The shoe is intended to permit lots of mobility in the feet and offer little cushioning, yet provide basic protection for lifting. The shoe's basic design is likened to that of other minimalistic footwear shoes such as the Vibram® 5 Fingers®. Over the past decade, the Reebok X-Company shoe has expanded to over six different variants for men and women (http://shop.reebok.com/us/shoes-X-Company/_/N-svZ1z12xfw) with each shoe reportedly offering differing support, lacing, and colors. The prices for these shoes start at roughly $99 a pair.

Forbes descried the partnership between Rebook® and X-Company as a way to solidify X-Company's commercial acceptance and potential for future investment. The actual monetized gains from the apparel and television exposure is unknown, but is likely significant in branding and new market acquisition. At the time of writing, X-Company did not have intentions of going public but certainly maintained that its numbers continued to grow. The Internet is chock-full of guides and forums to help a person open his or her own X-Company box. It seems that a new American entrepreneurial spirit may lie within a X-Company business.

So if at this point you are wondering if I've written a book about X-Company because I'm jealous of its financial success, I want you to know that this is far from the truth. The truth is that the fitness industry has seen its shares of gimmicks, fads, and devices. From trainers who take online certifications to electric devices that shock you into having a six-pack, the fitness world has struggled at exuding intelligent and honest works. Large, reputable organizations such as the American College of Sports Medicine and the National Strength and Conditioning Association have made significant efforts to rein in educating exercise specialists and provide national guidelines for healthy and unhealthy individuals. X-Company is not the answer to our fitness industry woes—it is just another problem, started by just another company.

The strength of any company is the composite of the knowledge, skills, and abilities of its people. With such outstanding revenue and potential profit, one would assume X-Company has a list of skilled affiliate trainers that "deliver" the service called "X-Company." Who are these trainers and what are their backgrounds? Read on to discover the shocking truth about their education and training.

Training the Trainer

During my X-Company "assessment," my trainer, who was certified through X-Company Inc., offered me new insights into the education and training of X-Company trainers. My trainer appeared to be in his late twenties or early thirties and very muscular. He had been doing X-Company for nearly four years after a military friend of his from California introduced him to the routine. At the end of my assessment I asked him if X-Company training was his full-time job and if he did X-Company himself. He remarked that he was a part-time trainer and was working another job in procuring vegetable oil from restaurants to make biodiesel. He also said that he no longer did X-Company—he had injured both shoulders, with one requiring surgery. As a result he focused on doing basic Olympic lifts for his training. I thought it nearly impossible that a person, especially someone with serious training goals or health issues, could be successful and safe with a part-time trainer who was not fully dedicated to his trade; moreover, this particular trainer injured himself while doing X-Company—how could he protect you? You might argue that certified trainer, whether full time or part time, may be all you need to get fit—but before you jump to conclusions, let's review the facts and the education and training of the many exercise specialists, including X-Company trainers.

Lon Kilgor, PhD, and X-Company founder Greg Glassman both have something to hold against the fitness industry: the lack of "practically" trained exercise specialists (http://library.crossfit.com/free/pdf/70_08_certifiable_knowledge.pdf). Published in the X-Company "journal," Lon writes on how the majority of exercise specialists (e.g., personal trainers, fitness specialists, strength coaches) do not have sufficient practical, or hands-on, training. He articulates that exercise specialists spend an exorbitant amount of time learning useless knowledge-based skills. Moreover, Lon feels the exercise specialist should not dabble in the clinical aspects of exercise. The clinical aspect of exercise is the study of advanced physiology of how exercise can be used in the treatment and prevention of diseases. Clinical exercise covers how exercise can be therapeutic and not simply for performance or aesthetic gains.

Clinical exercise is indeed a special area within the field of exercise science. Specialists who work in this area help patients regain strength, prevent further disease progression, and achieve goals despite major medical issues. Clinical exercise science requires in-depth physiological knowledge, advanced assessment and intervention techniques, and focused monitoring of clients. In many regards, clinical exercise science can be similar to physical therapy, only with clinical exercise having the goal of achieving more than rehabilitation for one focused injury or illness.

Lon's argument is outrageous that exercise specialists need to avoid the clinical components of exercise. In his article he cites that these clinical components provide little to the exercise specialist or client. I can agree partly with Lon in that some of the more basic clinical tests of balance or manual muscle testing in advanced athletes often are not rigorous enough to show deficits or change over time. In other words, athletes may have dysfunction or pain but the cause of these issues will not show with these basic tests—athletes and fit people need more rigorous, challenging tests. Certified athletic trainers and strength and conditioning specialists are trained in the knowledge and application of sport-specific testing and advanced methods for revealing performance deficits. Furthermore, physical therapists have extensive knowledge and practical training in assessing sport-specific deficits as they relate to clinical pathologies and functional deficits—particularly those physical therapists with board certifications in sports physical therapy.

Certified athletic trainers and strength and conditioning specialists and physical therapists all require a specific educational curriculum in order to obtain certification and/or licensing.

CERTIFIED ATHLETIC TRAINERS AND STRENGTH AND CONDITIONING SPECIALISTS:

- They are both trained in the knowledge and application of sport-specific testing and advanced methods for revealing performance deficits.

- Athletic training students, in order to sit for the entry-level board exam, must first graduate from an accredited program.

- Strength and conditioning students must also graduate from an exercise science program, although it is not stipulated (currently) for it to be accredited.

- Athletic training and strength and conditioning degrees are at the minimum of an associate's level, although nearly 75 percent of these individuals have a master's degree or higher.

PHYSICAL THERAPISTS:

- They must have extensive knowledge and practical training in assessing sport-specific deficits as they relate to clinical pathologies and functional deficits—particularly those physical therapists with board certifications in sports physical therapy.

- In order to sit for the entry-level board exam, they must first graduate from an accredited program.

- The entry-level physical therapist in the United States is now expected to obtain a doctoral-level degree in order to sit for the board examination.

- On the horizon, physical therapists may further be asked to enter into residencies, similar to other doctors like podiatrists and dentists, in order to practice.

We shall see what evolves over the next five to seven years. Regardless, these professions all maintain high academic rigor.

Lon is a professor at University of the West of Scotland in the Department of Anatomy and Physiology. As the program leader for Health Fitness Practice in this department, he should be very familiar with the training of exercise science students in most major universities within the United States. Exercise science programs require students to have not only book knowledge but also hands-on practical knowledge in order to pass what are known as "practical examinations." These examinations test the ability of the student in performing a specific exercise or rehabilitation-specific test or intervention. For instance, in a practical exam a strength and conditioning student must demonstrate and teach a person how to perform an Olympic lift. Or a physical therapy student must show how to properly manipulate a person's back during a spell of lower back pain. Practical examinations can be used as gatekeepers, preventing "weak-performing students from entering the internship phases of these programs.

The exercise science, athletic training, and physical therapy programs all require internships for their students. Athletic training and physical therapy students must meet a set number of internship hours under set criteria specified by an accrediting body. I know these standards as I used to teach across all three of these programs at Florida Gulf Coast University.

The programs discussed are the top-tiered exercise specialties in the United States. We did not discuss specialties such as occupational therapy, master-level clinical exercise physiologists, and others. However, it can be well documented that these exercise specialists have thorough education and expansive practical training, and are backed by large, vetted professional organizations. The beauty, but sometimes confusing bit, for consumers is where these people work after they graduate. These professional can work in a multitude of settings and obtain several additional certificates and specialties. The bottom line is that consumers should engage their exercise professionals to detail the settings they have worked in, the clientele they have worked with, and what specialties they hold—not all degrees and credentials are equal.

TV's *The Biggest Loser* has shown America how personal trainers can help obese individuals lose weight and gain better health through proper diet and exercise. One thing it does not elucidate is another concept that many consumers do no grasp: many personal trainers have limited educational and practical training. It is in this capacity that I agree with Lon Kilgore and Greg Glassman—the below-average to average personal trainer who took a weekend course in training does not have the practical skills to guide you in exercise. The industry for certifying these individuals is massive, especially with certificates costing about $200 and many of the certificates being delivered online. The online delivery makes it easy to pass (with multiple attempts permitted in some cases) and very affordable to the company offering the exam, thus maximizing the profits of the certifying organization or company. The majority of these examinations cover basic exercise testing, prescription, and safety knowledge—no hands-on training is involved. Most of my exercise- and rehab-related colleagues and I have major issues with these rogue organizations.

The certificate holders from these organizations often do the job of cleaning machines, filing papers, and the occasional task of personal training at the large box gyms. Publications have shown that many for-profit education institutes have targeted returning GIs, who can obtain funding for education through the GI Bill, as they returned from Iraq and Afghanistan (http://abcnews.go.com/Business/president-obama-signs-executive-order-protecting-veter-ans-inundated/story?id=16219870). The allure of making big bucks from personal training with minimal effort, all at the expense of the taxpayer, seems lucrative. However, it is sad to say few make it through the for-profit school programs (roughly 60 percent default on their loans); those who do pass the programs are minimally motivated to learn beyond the basics, are entrenched in nonresearched based methods, and embrace exercise as a glamor tool for looking good. Only a few of these individuals excel in their postcertificate education. These GIs struggle because the nonaccredited for-profit educational institutions have let them down. Without proper educational accreditation and with the need to maximize student enrollment, students are left with a poor education and training that does more harm than good.

These GIs struggle because the nonaccredited for-profit educational institutions have let them down. Without proper educational accreditation and with the need to maximize student enrollment, students are left with a poor education and training that does more harm than good.

Where does X-Company stand with these organizations? X-Company is no different than the rogue organization that offers a basic certificate for training over the course of weekend. X-Company does not have a professional organization that mandates educational competencies or accreditation. Furthermore, no prerequisites are needed to attend the weekend course, with the exception of being older than seventeen years of age. In order to sit for the exam, the applicant must attend the entire weekend course, participate in the "practical sections," and pass the Level 1 exam in person. X-Company trainers are no different than the trainers who take online courses, although they are exposed to some movements, such as Olympic lifting and the common X-Company moves in a physical classroom setting. I would argue, along with many of my strength and conditioning friends, that Olympic lifts are far from basic and should not be included in the most rudimentary training certificate course. But this is X-Company and everything is extreme, right?

The cost for a weekend X-Company Level 1 course is $1,000. A portion of this money goes to the "box" offering the course; meanwhile, the remainder is sent to X-Company Inc. The company provides the trainer's handbook (http://www.cross-fit.com/ cf-seminars/ CertRefs/CFD_L1_ParticipantHandbook_Revised_02.pdf), which was created by Greg Glassman and has been updated by his company's "Certification and Training Department."

The Level 1 course serves as an introduction to X-Company and to meet these goals:

1. Provide attendees an understanding of how to use X-Company for themselves

2. Provide attendees an initial and foundational understanding of X-Company in order to train others

In short, the main goals are to introduce soon-to-be trainers on how to use X-Company themselves and provide a basic understanding of what X-Company is, in order to begin training others. It would seem that you would want further depth in the goals of a course, other than an introduction, before you allowed individuals to begin training others. Recall, these Level 1 trainers, after passing the exam, are permitted to train individuals on their own, without the requirement of guidance from more senior members. My trainer during my assessment was a Level 1 trainer. Also, don't forget that this Level 1 certification is required in order to open a gym—so consumer beware; if a new box opens near you, the instructor may be a newbie.

The trainer's handbook goes further with the Level 1 certification through established educational objectives:

- Define the core concepts of the X-Company program
- Identify the primary points of performance of the foundational movements
- Perform the foundational movements safely and identify when they have a violation of sound movement
- Identify correct movement when training others
- Identify violations of sound movement and apply appropriate correction toward improved movement
- Apply the X-Company program safely and effectively, while gaining experience necessary to develop competency in other X-Company training methods

The objectives listed have some major flaws.

First, the objectives listed may be challenging, if not impossible, to measure. For instance, how do you measure that a person can apply the X-Company program safely and effectively? Will the evaluators follow those who have been trained by a Level 1 trainer to ensure a X-Company program meets their fitness needs and has not caused harm? This scenario is unlikely as it would be time-consuming and challenging to measure, particularly as people often travel to large cities to sit for their exams. This scenario is very feasible in the educational internship setting where a clinical instructor can assess how a student treats a cohort of clients over a period of time.

Second, if this is an introduction to exercise, where are the foundational principles of exercise physiology, or even normal physiology for that matter? Again, X-Company presents itself as irreverent to scientific principles and well-tested principles—even in its education for its trainers. Moreover, some of the individuals taking the Level 1 course have never exercised or at least have not touched much of the high-intensity exercise equipment. Equipment such as Olympic bars, rings, and parallel bars can be very dangerous during exercise, especially if the trainer is not educated in the basic safety needs of this equipment.

An example of the possible lack of basic safety training is the unfortunate incident of Kevin Ogar—he severed his spinal cord while competing in a X-Company tournament. You can view the video of Kevin's accident online (http://www.liveleak.com/view?i=d5c _1389972271). In the beginning video you can see that Kevin, a X-Company trainer himself, was beginning his lift slightly too far back on the lifting platform (large rubber mats where the athlete stands). On the left of the screen you can see another X-Company trainer/official supervising Kevin's lift.

Behind Kevin you can clearly see a stack of weights that are abutting the lifting platform. It is basic safety knowledge in the strength and conditioning educational programs that stacking excessive weights too close to a lifting platform can be dangerous. How did the seasoned X-Company official and Kevin, the X-Company trainer, not recognize Kevin's poor setup on the platform and the dangerous stack of weights? Were they not educated on these basic safety practices?

Third, foundational movements are important but are not applicable in every training situation. For instance, a X-Company trainer, in an online video of a Level 1 course evaluation, remarks that squatting is a basic movement we all must do (http://journal. crossfit.com/2009/01/the-level-2-cert-a-simulated-test-1.tpl). I can agree with this notion, as I often use squats with many of my clients for various health- and performance-related goals (e.g., building bones, improving strength, losing weight, improve transfers). However, despite my love for squats and how basic a move it is, not all clients are well suited for squats. Furthermore, not all programs need squats if other exercises are included or the goals of the movements far exceed the basic movement of squatting.

A good example of these two issues would be a person who has a bad tracking kneecap (patellofemoral pain syndrome). Squatting can be painful and sometimes not appropriate in an acute phase. In an instance where squatting may be too basic, consider a football lineman. Having him perform basic squats does not prepare him to sufficiently explode into another lineman—this is where power exercises (e.g., cleans or deadlifts) are appropriate. We will discuss an important athlete training concept called periodized training later, but suffice it to say that squats are not always appropriate. No core group of exercises are appropriate for all people—this is a reductionist view that merely facilitates easy exercise programming for the trainer and maintains employment of poorly trained "exercise" personnel by limiting their creativity and expansion into other training modalities. My X-Company trainer had me completing deep knee squats during my assessment despite my knee injury and surgery. Of course he did not know about my knee injury because he never asked and the facility never had me list my medical/health history. I did mention my knee issue to him—his remarks were that my form was fine and to continue as long as it didn't hurt. At the time of doing the squat, my knee was fine—the next day my knee was sore, which was something I had not felt in years (and I am ranked "good" for lower body strength, leg pressing nearly four hundred pounds without knee pain three times per week). I could see how someone could easily get sore because a trainer and organization were forcing a general routine onto everyone.

Fourth, the last objective makes it clear that the goal of X-Company's Level 1 course is to get you hooked and keep you coming back for more classes. True educational leaders in exercise science and physical therapy promote their students to blossom into a varied educational setting and medium. Specialization may be important, but education comes from many sources.

X-Company escalates its educational scheme with the X-Company Coach's Prep course (http://www.crossfit.com/cf-info/certs.shtml). The Coach's Prep course covers additional programming topics and further builds on the foundations in the Level 1 course.

Many consider the Coach's Prep course an intermediate course for those interested in going from Level 1 to Level 2 certification. Fabio Comana, MS, MA, of the American Council of Exercise (ACE), summarized the Level 1 and Coach's Prep courses as "remedial when one considers the nature and intensity of the exercises performed" (http://www.acefitness.org/ certifiednewsarticle/962/crossfit-is-the-gain-worth-the-pain-ace-experts). Mr. Comana further said that the Level 2 course is where X-Company trainers advance their education and practical knowledge to nearly the level of a strength and conditioning coach. The key word is nearly.

The Level 2 certification covers the nine core movements of X-Company: the front squat, back squat, overhead squat, sumo-squat to high-pull, push press, press, pull jerk, deadlift, and clean (http://journal.crossfit.com/2009/02/the-level-2-cert-a-simulated-test-2--- the-evaluation.tpl). A couple of these movements are essential for strengthening of the legs across all populations; however, again, the movements of the clean and push press are power-based movements. Power-based movements involve explosive muscle contractions that use almost the entire body. Power-based movements require a substantial base of strength, along with proper coordination and mechanics in order to prevent injury. This does not mean that all power-based movements are inappropriate for the nonathletic populations. We will discuss the importance of power-based movements and their appropriateness in a later section. Regardless, the fact these explosive movements are the bedrock for the educational competency of X-Company shows the obvious bias toward power training. X-Company trainers are losing the opportunity to learn other modes of resistance training, flexibility work, and balance concepts due to this bias. Keep in mind these trainers are being prepared to "scale" their workouts for anyone, or in the X-Company lingo, "any kind." ABC News recently published a report on X-Company Kids (http://abcnews.go.com/blogs/ health/2013/11/06/is-crossfit-training-safe-for-children/). X-Company Kids is the same exercise program done by adults only "scaled" or made easier for kids. The article highlights a sports medicine physician with obvious reservations about the program; however, one thing was missing: no one questioned whether the X-Company staff had the educational competency to work with a developing population.

Exercise must be adapted according to lifespan development. Certain exercise can either or hinder or improve a person's wellness depending on the person's age and development. For instance, an older adult will need to focus extensively on training the strength of the hips, thighs, calves, while addressing balance and flexibility. The focus of these exercises is to prevent age-related muscle mass loss, prevent falls, and maintain mobility. On the other hand, a younger adolescent may need to have his or her exercise focus on speed, cutting, and cardiovascular exercise for sport and obesity prevention. The exercise specialist adapts the program to the specific person taking into consideration his or her chronological age and the duration/experience with training.

The concept of exercise and aging across the lifespan is a bedrock educational objective among exercise science and physical therapy programs. A review of its core educational objectives (in the handbook) shows that X-Company Inc. does not prepare the X-Company trainer for training a developing child.

Without having a well-rounded curriculum regarding human movement and physiology, X-Company trainers may be walking away with little more than a piece a paper and a sore back—and you or your child may be their next victim.

IN SUMMARY:

• The ACSM has put forth safe ways for many populations to exercise. Visit www.acsm.org for more information regarding exercise position statements for pregnancy, illnesses, and general wellness.

• X-Company Inc. does not accredit, inspect, or measure the success of these affiliate gyms. As such, the only requirement for a box to begin and continue to educate new trainers every year is money.

• Gross revenue for 2012 was estimated to be well over $20 million.

• X-Company does not adequately screen or review exercisers' medical history—this increases the risk for injury or death and violates many standard exercise guidelines.

• X-Company's "journal" is not peer-reviewed or refereed. It lacks scientific rigor and does not publish quality studies or trials.

• X-Company trainers do not have sufficient education or practical training to work with unhealthy populations, let alone healthy populations.

• X-Company does not educate its staff on lifespan health issues and clinical exercise science principles.

• X-Company does not have training guidelines for the different needs of clients based on age or clinical needs.

• If you feel the need to try X-Company, consider exercising with a personal trainer first. Be sure he or she takes your medical history, performs a baseline assessment, frequently checks your exercise intensity by taking your heart rate or perceived effort, and modifies your program if you have pain or problems.

• Select an exercise or fitness specialist who has a minimum of a bachelor's degree in exercise science, athletic training, human performance, kinesiology, or premedicine. These individuals have the physiological and applied backgrounds to help you the most.

Chapter 4: Uncle Rhabdo and How I Learned to Stop Worrying and Love the Burn

"My elbows were stuck in a bent position—I couldn't straighten my arms. I texted my CrossFit Trainer—she told me to come back to the box for another workout as it would help my soreness …It turned out I had rhabdo…"

—From an interview with a Southwest Florida businessman who developed rhabdo.

Have you ever seen a picture of a clown attached to a dialysis machine with his kidney and guts hanging out? If you haven't, perhaps you missed the rhabdomyolysis educational campaign promoted by the "head trainer" of X-Company, Russell Berger. Mr. Berger found himself answering several questions after a colleague of mine from Regis University published a scathing article regarding "X-Company's Dirty Little Secret": rhabdomyolysis (http://www.huffington post.com/eric-robertson/crossfit-rhabdomyolysis_b_3977598.html).

Rhabdomyolysis is a serious medical condition. It involves a full-body breakdown of the proteins in your body, particularly muscle tissue. Several conditions and diseases can cause rhabdomyolysis, jokingly called "Uncle Rhabdo" in the

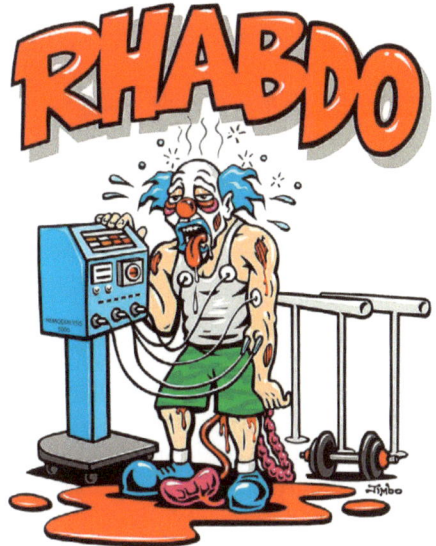

"Uncle Rhabdo" (from www.crossfit.com)

X-Company world. In the case of X-Company, rhabdo occurs because of overexertion.

In short, the proteins in the muscles explode into the bloodstream. This can result in kidney failure, heart abnormalities, and even death in roughly 5 percent of cases (Joshua Latham, Darren Campbell, and William Nichols. "How much exercise can raise creatine kinase levels?" Journal of Family Practice. 2008). X-Company's response to this serious medical condition was to create a cute clown picture to put in its journal, on its website, and on T-shirts.

I was amazed at the number of people I encountered while writing this book that suffered from X-Company-induced rhabdo. The incidents ranged from personal accounts of a friend's boss to a very fit triathlete—X-Company's ugly side effect was having a significant impact on my friends and neighbors. The stories of these individuals are shocking yet enlightening.

In this chapter we will explore rhabdo, how it happens, and the actual exercise behind X-Company. We will examine the intensity of the workouts, look at how exercise is reportedly "scaled," and analyze how the exercise is progressed. Understanding these factors can help you prevent rhabdo and other chronic musculoskeletal injuries.

X-Company-Induced Rhabdo

Mr. Berger, the head trainer for X-Company, stated during an interview with ABC News on September 26, 2013, "We have articles in X-Company journal when we first learned about exercise-induced rhabdo" (http://abcnews.go.com/health/2013/09/26/crossfit-can-the-popular-extreme-workout-be-dangerous/). Furthermore, he commented on how the clown, despite the fact that it is grotesque, brings awareness to the topic of rhabdomyolysis.

Recall that Greg Glassman established X-Company in 2003. Despite nearly ten years of operating, his head trainer admits to the public that they finally "learned about exercise-induced rhabdo." Glassman wrote an article in his X-Company journal titled "X-Company Induced Rhabdo" in October 2005, two years after establishing X-Company (http://journal.crossfit.com/2005/10/X-Company-induced-rhabdo-by-gre.tpl). In this article, Glassman does not recommend the monitoring of intensity through heart rate measures. Nor does he cite the need to use evidenced-based intensity scales such as the Borg Intensity Scale. Glassman actually brags about X-Company's "potency."

The fact that rhabdo was not apparent to X-Company trainers, the founder, or X-Company's many departments reinforces the lack of human physiological understanding that X-Company personnel have; furthermore, it underscores how the X-Company organization may have been myopic and resistant to see a major side effect from their training as an "issue" until years later. Glassman reports on his website blog on October 2005 that five individuals suffered from exertional rhabdo due to X-Company. Again, Glassman, the founder and beneficiary of X-Company Inc., reported only 5 incidents of exertional rhabdo due to X-Company. In 2005 Glassman had only thirteen facilities; it's been almost a decade since then and X-Company has grown to seven thousand facilities. What exactly is the prevalence of rhabdo in exercise and X-Company? One could, based on this growth relative to the number of people with rhabdo in 2005, estimate that 2,692 people experienced X-Company-induced rhabdo in 2013. Of course, this is a very rough estimate based solely on the number of people with rhabdo and the growth of the company. Other variables likely have an impact on these data.

Had more academics been involved, or if the organizational structure were founded on professional ideals, X-Company case studies and reports would have been published in national peer-reviewed journals. Publications in such large objective journals would have exposed X-Company's educational weaknesses and promoted safe exercise and program modifications before others became exposed to potential injury. Recall that X-Company Inc. owns the rhabdo educational material in X-Company's journal—why publish damning information about your business in a national journal when you can contain the public relations nightmare to your own "newsletter" journal?

Business aside, rhabdo can kill and the X-Company exercise regimen may be at fault. Dr. Robertson from Regis University highlighted how a fellow physical therapist succumbed to rhabdo following a X-Company training session. Jill Kloesel apparently had no warning signs of rhabdo. After her X-Company session, her arms swelled significantly and she admitted herself to the emergency department. In the emergency department her creatine phosphokinase (CPK) levels were so high that they could not be reported. CPK testing checks the level of muscle protein, or myoglobin, that is in the blood. It is this myoglobin, which is stocked with nitrogen, that can seriously damage your kidneys. Jill spent five days in the intensive care unit in order to recover from her X-Company workout. Another person who spent several days in the hospital was a gentleman from Southwest Florida who had been doing X-Company for over a year. This gentleman has asked to remain anonymous, so we will call him "John." John has years of experience with training and exercise. Unfortunately, exercise experience proved to be useless in order to safely engage in X-Company.

John detailed the workout of the day (WOD) from his last X-Company session: as many pull-ups possible alternated by a 400-meter sprint, cycled as many times possible for twenty minutes. John thought the workout to be challenging, but nothing he wasn't up for. He loved the challenge and intensity of X-Company—it allowed him to think of nothing but surviving the exercise routine—it was an escape from work and life. John finished this workout on a Monday night in December. He was slightly dehydrated, but he quickly replenished his fluids that night.

John woke up the next morning sore, stiff, and oddly tired. He had no major pains but felt "odd." He thought about returning to the box for another workout on Tuesday but he was exhausted—he was in bed by 7:00 p.m. John described the scary scene he faced Wednesday morning when he woke up:

"My elbows were stuck in a bent position—I couldn't straighten my arms. My son tried to straighten my arms: the pain wasn't ten out of ten—it was twenty out of ten. I texted my X-Company trainer—she told me to come back to the box for another workout as it would help my soreness."

John was wise to not return to the gym; instead, he gingerly dressed himself with help from family, and he went into the office. His wife thought he should seek medical care— John thought it useless as many medical doctors know so little about exercise and training. It was that afternoon when his urine turned to the color of cola. His wife, being concerned when his condition did not resolve Wednesday night, investigated on the Internet all the potential causes of John's muscle soreness and urine discoloration. She found a website detailing rhabdo, its signs and symptoms, and treatment course. After learning that rhabdo can kill your kidneys, John decided to admit himself to the local hospital. His CPK levels hit 86,000—that is nearly 1,433 percent higher than a normal, healthy range.

Fortunately, his kidneys were fine, but the medical staff held him for monitoring for seven days. After copious saline, medicines, and monitoring, John luckily survived his exposure to X-Company-induced rhabdo, but at what cost? He had thousands of dollars in medical bills and lost time from work, and he continues to have muscle weakness in his arms. Nearly two months later, he still struggles to hold his newborn six-pound baby.

The Research

The direct link between exercise and rhabdo is not new. Rhabdo does not only happen in X-Company settings. As Mr. Berger, the head X-Company trainer, cited in his ABC interview, "There are cases of rhabdo from football players, people who run triathlons, marathon runners to military trainees to body-building communities." Many of these cases were published in national, peer-reviewed journals or published at yearly professional conventions. The benefit of this publication and discussion is that as a result of this process, professionals educate professionals and develop a plan for prevention and treatment, if necessary.

I researched when and how the first X-Company induced rhabdo case occurred— unfortunately this data is not publicly available. I did find intriguing comments written in 2007 in response to Greg Glassman's X-Company-induced rhabdo article I mentioned above. The comments are frankly sad, with many of the people saying that they wished they had known the risk of developing rhabdo before beginning X-Company. Several mentioned that they found themselves hospitalized for three to five days and practically unable to move. Most of the people injured stated they were "fit" and routine exercisers. You can view these comments here: http://journal.crossfit.com/2005/10/X-Company-induced-rhabdo-by-gre.tpl.

Fortunately, I did not experience rhabdo with my X-Company experience. My fitness status would be considered excellent to very good for most fitness functions, according to the ACSM. I exercise for nearly forty-five minutes six days per week, performing strengthening, explosive and balance movements, cardiovascular exercises, and stretching. Despite this training, X-Company was still challenging for me—I can only imagine what it would be like for an "average Joe" walking off the street, especially if he had health issues. The assessment, which was "standard" for X-Company according to my trainer, involved a 500-meter row on a rowing machine, forty deep squats without weights, thirty sit-ups, twenty push-ups, and ten pull-ups. My trainer remarked that an "excellent" X-Company exercisers could do all of this in five minutes but that most newbies did it ten minutes. I finished the assessment in seven minutes and was exhausted. I routinely can perform fifty to sixty push-ups—I could barely do ten push-ups without stopping. Why was it so hard for me? It comes down to simple physiology, energy, and rest—the physiology being the least studied and measured in the X-Company arena. My heart rate, taken by me and not by my trainer, measured at 186 beats per minute, which exceeds my maximum heart rate. Had my trainer measured my intensity using a scale or heart rate device, he could have guided me to rest longer, which may have helped me finish the routine better and without sacrificing form or risking injury.

Rhabdo's History

Exercise-induced rhabdo is not a new phenomenon. In 1974 in the Archives of Internal Medicine, several authors published an article focusing on exercise-induced rhabdo in exercising Marines. The number of reported cases in non-X-Company settings is fairly low. In a large six-year study in Taiwan, researchers looked back at the number children and adolescences (eighteen years old and younger) reporting to the emergency department with diagnosed rhabdo (Chun-Yu Chen et al. "Clinical spectrum of rhabdomyolysis presented to pediatric emergency department." BMC Pediatrics 13.1 [2013]: 134). Of the 165,000 children and adolescences that physicians examined, thirty-seven had the diagnosis of rhabdo. Out of thirty-seven of these subjects, only six had the diagnosis of exercise-induced rhabdo. This is 6/165,000 children (in Taiwan) admitted to the emergency room—this does not factor in those children or adolescences who did not present to the emergency room or adults with rhabdo.

In another retrospective study, physicians admitted 250,000 people in the time period of 1988–1993 to a hospital. Of these adults, they diagnosed thirty-five adults with exercise induced-rhabdo. This is slightly higher than the Taiwanese study; however, the number of those admitted for exercise-induced rhabdo remains quite low.

When looking at the multiple case studies that have been published, it is obvious that many cases occur in military, firefighter, and police officer training. A 2005 article that stands out from the pack is Lin, Lin, Wang, and Leu's short report (http://www.bjsportmed.com/cgi/content/full/39/1/e3; doi: 10.1136/bjsm.2004.013235). These authors published an article in the British Journal of Sports Medicine on exercise-induced rhabdo in high school students. In the report, the authors wrote that the children were tasked by their gymnastic teacher to perform 120 push-ups in five minutes—a very similar task that you might see in X-Company facility. All 119 kids developed exercise-induced rhabdo and need further treatment in an emergency department. It is one thing for a soldier or police officer to suffer from overtraining, but is X-Company-style exercise really appropriate for kids, let alone anyone in the normal population? To answer this question and others, let's look at how the exercise is reportedly measured and progressed.

The Exercise Intensity, Scaling, and Progression

Power-based movements are explosive movements that help an athlete to improve speed. The correct use, according to the NSCA, of power-based movements involves few repetitions but with very heavy weight at very fast speeds. More importantly, the weight used during these movements is very specific to the individual lifter—this helps him maximize his gains and reduce the likelihood of injury. X-Company does not individualize the weight lifting through proper maximum weight assessments; moreover, X-Company frequently uses a very high number of repetitions despite the weight being light or heavy. It is this injudicious use of high repetitions that significantly increases the likelihood of injury for the X-Company exercisers. Power-based movements started with athletes and are used successfully with a large majority of sports teams. The movements are fast and help athletes move more quickly. Additionally, power-based movements have been shown to be safe for athletes. What about you, the nonathlete? What about your mother, the kind seventy-year-old woman with a bad back? Are power-based movements safe for either of you?

Luckily we have had several bright exercise scientists demonstrate the safety of power-based training, following NSCA guidelines, in the elderly and in special populations (Tim R. Henwood, Stephan Riek, and Dennis R. Taaffe. "Strength versus muscle power-specific resistance training in community-dwelling older adults." The Journals of Gerontology Series A: Biological Sciences and Medical Sciences 63.1 [2008]: 83–91. Rhonda Orr et al. "Power training improves balance in healthy older adults." The Journals of Gerontology Series A: Biological Sciences and Medical Sciences 61.1 [2006]: 78–85). Where are the published studies of the safety of X-Company moves for these same populations? **The answer will not surprise you: there are none.**

Now that we have addressed that these power-based movements following NSCA guidelines can be safe in older and special populations, let's address why a person might use these training techniques in nonathletes. After all, why would my eighty-year-old grandfather want to gain speed, right? Consider this notion: when people fall, they fall quickly. Older adults are prone to lose their balance due to myriad reasons such as reduced strength, reduced power, poor neuromuscular control, and so on. While many of these factors seem important, it is vital to see the difference between power and strength:

- Power is the ability to apply a large force as quickly as possible.

- Strength is simply the amount of force you can exert.

Therefore, to keep someone from falling, exercise specialists need to focus on power training, not simply strength training. Power training is no longer reserved for athletes, but there are several prerequisites that are needed before a person begins to power train.

In the field of exercise science and sports training, exercise specialists pay close attention to several factors of intensity to prevent injury and maximize performance gains. The most commonly measured factors of intensity are the weight of the lift, heart rate, the speed of the lift, the volume of exercise (number of total lifts multiplied by the weight lifted), and the complexity of the movement (e.g., many joints, one joint, high-level coordination required). Intensity can produce results but can easily produce injuries; thus, it is vital that intensity is closely monitored.

Several online forums (Catalyst, Bodybuilding.com) have posts from regular exercisers that attempted X-Company. The intensity was so high that many of these fit individuals reported the inability to move their arms, legs, or entire body for nearly a week. Several cited that this was even after the WOD (X-Company's workout of the day) was "scaled." X-Company exercisers on the forum rebutted, saying that the symptoms were merely delayed onset muscle soreness, or DOMS. DOMS, according to the American College of Sports Medicine, is muscle soreness that occurs twelve to twenty-four hours after exercise and lasts for only three to five days (http://www.acsm.org/docs/brochures/delayed-onset-muscle-soreness-%28doms%29.pdf). It is obvious that the people in pain were likely suffering from rhabdomyolysis, and that the rebutting X-Company exercisers were not well-versed on DOMS let alone rhabdo. Again, these posts were from "fit" people—imagine what would happen if you were unfit or not physically active at all?

I had the opportunity to interview a South Florida bartender who injured himself during X-Company. He had been exercising for years before trying X-Company, performing both strengthening and cardiovascular exercises. His routine of the usual dumbbells and machines bored him, so he decided to check out an exercise program that many of his friends raved about—this routine was X-Company.

After the first session of X-Company, he knew he found the program to push him aggressively and change his routine—exactly what he wanted. At first most of the exercises were similar to what he had been doing, but they were more intense or slightly more complicated. However, by the fourth session the X-Company trainers had progressed him to performing Olympic lifts over his head. In the strength and conditioning profession, these exercises take months, if not years, to master. X-Company progressed him to performing these lifts in only four sessions, which took place in less than a month! It is no surprise that this fit young man began to develop neck and lower back pain.

After seeking care from a licensed massage therapist, his neck pain resolved. He wavered on returning to X-Company because he felt the X-Company trainers had accelerated his progression too quickly and did not provide him the guidance he needed for such advanced exercises. In reality his progression was on par with the normal progression for exercises for X-Company—my X-Company trainer also wanted me to perform overhead Olympic lifts by the fourth session. You can view how dangerous these exercises can become when performed by novice X-Company exercisers here:

http://www.youtube.com/watch?v=M8up6A4QesU&feature=player_embedded&desktop_uri=%2Fwatch%3Ffeature%3Dplayer_embedded&app=desktop.

This bartender's opinion validates the many doubts this book posits in that X-Company does not offer the appropriate supervision and coaching for such a high-intensity exercise program. He loved the camaraderie and push of X-Company, although he does feel it is like a "cult." He has returned to doing his own version of X-Company-style exercise at his local gym and has yet to have neck or back pain since.

Intensity Bottom Line

The X-Company culture does not measure intensity in the same fashion as exercise scientists. Recall that X-Company is a high-intensity, constantly varied exercise routine. As such, the X-Company culture has accepted that the exercise routine is supposed to be of high intensity. **X-Company exercisers do not monitor their heart rates, do not track their volume of exercise between sessions, and almost always use complex/large movements for their exercise** (which are naturally more intensive). Granted, X-Company exercisers do track their weight lifted and time each other to complete movements, but these metrics are geared to measuring performance and not ensuring safety.

So how can anyone perform X-Company and not get injured? The X-Company journal and X-Company trainers point to one word: **scaling**.

Weighing the Scales

Scaling is the term used in X-Company that describes how exercise intensity is adapted to match the fitness level of a person. In the world of exercise science, scaling is known as exercise prescription. Physical therapists may refer to it as "dosing." It is important to note that X-Company's term does not have the same meaning as that of exercise scientists and physical therapists. Scaling does not exactly equate to a change in exercise prescription or dosing—several differences exist and will be explained below.

First, scaling does not modify all of the components of exercise intensity. For instance, if a person begins to perform a lift and her form is poor, the first response for scaling would be to lower the weight. An exercise scientist may also consider lowering the weight to be the first option. A physical therapist may also consider that the person who has poor form during a lift may not have the motor control (combination of coordination and muscle firing patterns) to perform the movement properly and safely. As such, the physical therapist may select a different exercise that a person can perform with good form, while still promoting the same muscles and performance enhancements. By choosing a different exercise, the physical therapist is modifying another component of exercise intensity: the mode or type of exercise. With X-Company's persistent bias toward large/gross movement patterns, it does not allow the exerciser the opportunity to attempt a more basic exercise that may be more appropriate and beneficial. A more basic exercise often is needed prior to performing larger movement patterns. Motor control principles and exercise progression concepts are covered thoroughly in exercise science and physical therapy educational programs.

The second issue with X-Company's scaling is that it makes the assumption that all the exercises done in X-Company are appropriate for all individuals. The notion that anyone can do X-Company is apparent across many major X-Company websites, in advertising, and within its cultural mantra. No well-educated and ethical exercise professional should make the claim that one exercise program is appropriate for all people, as this is fundamentally impossible. Again, it is X-Company's lack of education and accredited training for its trainers that puts X-Company exercisers at such a risk for injury.

The third issue with scaling is that it ignores assessment. When an exercise scientist or physical therapist prescribes/doses exercise, he or she performs an assessment prior to beginning exercise. It is this assessment that allows for the proper exercise and intensity selection. Moreover, the assessment ensures that no contraindications for exercise exist. Absolute contraindications are exercises or treatments that should not be performed because a client has certain diseases, conditions, or factors. The declaration of a contraindicated exercise comes from longitudinal studies, high-level research (usually groups or organizations that agree as a whole), or when there is too much risk for a small potential benefit. For instance, it is contraindicated for a pregnant woman to perform exercise if she is bleeding from her cervix (http://www.acog.org/~/media/For%20Patients/faq119.pdf). This example makes sense because the risk of losing the baby does not outweigh the benefit of the exercise. Moreover, research supports that this type of bleeding may be a sign that labor is near—exercise will only increase the rate of delivery, which may be premature. Absolute contraindications have legal ramifications. If a practitioner provides a treatment or exercise that is contraindicated, then that practitioner may be liable for any injuries he causes his clients related to that exercise. Therefore, it is important for exercise specialists to know these absolute contraindications.

Precautions, or relative contraindications, also exist. Precautions are different than contraindications in that precautions caution or urge clinicians to select other exercises or treatments due to a potential risk for injury in a selected population or person. Precautions have less legal teeth than absolute contraindications, as precautions are recommendations that often warrant a clinician's judgment at a particular time and circumstance. Precautions are similar to contraindications in that they are founded based on research, practice, and often a professional consensus. A common precaution in physical therapy is to not perform repetitive lower back bending if a person has lower back pain or history of a disc injury. In this example, the precaution does not completely stop a physical therapist from allowing a person to bend in their lower back. The client may have short-term relief of his lower back pain with bending in his lower back; however, it may be advantageous to the client's long-term health to not bend his lower back excessively during exercise if he has had lower back issues in the past (http://www.ideafit.com/fitness-library/the-painful-lumbar-spine).

The concern many exercise specialists have is that X-Company, along with many of the "weekend" personal trainers, have not had the depth or breadth of education regarding contraindications and precautions. This became starkly apparent after several pregnant women lifting very heavy weights during X-Company posted their pictures on social media. The American College of Gynecologists urges women to exercise but to limit the intensity to a moderate level. Why didn't the X-Company organization step in to show it does not condone this exercise approach? The answer is simple: the X-Company community has not been educated in these precautions (examine X-Company's trainer educational competencies). Precautions to exercise during pregnancy, such as muscle weakness, can often be ignored and "pushed" through, placing both the child and mother at risk. If scaling is the answer, how does X-Company know it has scaled the exercise appropriately for its client? Recall that X-Company trainers and exercisers do not routinely take heart rates, perceived exertion scale ratings, or other standardized forms of intensity assessments. Lastly, it should be stated that no scientific articles have been published in peer-reviewed journals regarding the safety of "scaled" X-Company for pregnant women; in fact, no peer-reviewed journal articles have been published on the effectiveness and safety of scaling in any population.

Progression or Regression?

Working in the field of exercise science and rehabilitation is extremely rewarding. From seeing a client achieve his or her first marathon to helping an older adult walk without a walker for the first time, the metamorphosis in body function and ability is amazing. Much of the positive change is not happenstance; rather, it is a result of planning, proper prescribing, and progressive overloading.

Overloading is the progressive increase in exercise intensity in order to elicit a positive change in function. Typically, exercise specialists use overloading to increase muscular strength, but they can also use it to improve endurance, power, and even balance. Without overloading, athletes would never get faster, clients would stay at the same strength levels, and patients would never balance better. In order to see positive changes, the exercise program must safely push the client beyond the normal forces he or she experiences in a typical day. Anyone who has worked out before knows that it can be challenging to know when to lift more or when to back off. This decision may seem more like an art than a science, but sound science and guidelines do exist to guide clinicians in exercise progression.

The National Strength and Conditioning Association (NSCA) provides clear guidelines on progressing strengthening exercises. The two-for-two rule stipulates that if person is able to lift two additional repetitions on two subsequent workouts, the weight should be progressed for that exercise (Thomas R. Baechle and Roger W. Earle. Essentials of Strength Training and Conditioning. 2008: Human Kinetics). If the weight is not progressed, another exercise may be added that is similar or targets the same areas of the body. Adding another exercise increases volume of exercise, which increases the intensity of the workout.

Several peer-reviewed research articles have covered how an exercise specialist ought to change exercise volume and intensity of elite and high-intensity athletes (William J. Kraemer et al. "Influence of resistance training volume and periodization on physiological and performance adaptations in collegiate women tennis players." The American Journal of Sports Medicine 28.5 [2000]: 626–633; William J. Kraemer and Nicholas A. Ratamess. "Fundamentals of resistance training: progression and exercise prescription." Medicine and Science in Sports and Exercise 36.4 [2004]: 674–688). A large majority of these publications focus on a concept called periodization.

Periodization is training that is broken down into sections of time with planned changes in exercise intensity. It is important to note that these are planned changes in exercise volume and intensity—they are not variable, as in the case of X-Company. Studies show that the planning and tracking of exercise volume significantly reduce the rate of injury while maximizing performance gains (Timothy E. Hewett, Kevin R. Ford, and Gregory D. Myer. "Anterior cruciate ligament injuries in female athletes Part 2, a meta-analysis of neuromuscular interventions aimed at injury prevention." The American Journal of Sports Medicine 34.3 [2006]: 490–498; William J. Kraemer and Nicholas A. Ratamess. "Fundamentals of resistance training: progression and exercise prescription." Medicine and Science in Sports and Exercise 36.4 [2004]: 674–688).

The initial purpose of this style of training was to prepare athletes for an event or competitive season. Athletes would train at high volumes and at low to moderate intensity several months prior to competition, only to lower volume and increase intensity just before competition. During the season, the focus may be on merely maintaining strength, not increasing it, as this increases the risk for injury. When an athlete is injured it can be devastating, as the certified athletic trainer may have to pull the athlete from competition.

Because of the differing physical demands of each sport, every sport has a unique periodization plan. Over the past two decades, researchers considered that periodization training might not be just for athletes (Carmen Castaneda et al. "A randomized controlled trial of resistance exercise training to improve glycemic control in older adults with type 2 diabetes." Diabetes Care 25.12 [2002]: 2335–2341; David J. Kosek et al. "Efficacy of 3 days/wk resistance training on myofiber hypertrophy and myogenic mechanisms in young vs. older adults." Journal of Applied Physiology 101.2 [2006]: 531–544). As such, they began researching the effects of periodized training in the nonathlete. Much to the researchers' surprise, periodized training works for many individuals.

Periodized training for the nonathlete is safe and effective. Initially you might ask what events are these individuals training for considering they are not playing a sport? The answer is that periodized training ensures that a person does not overtrain, and it hones multiple areas of fitness. Periodized training can also prepare a person for recreation activities and sports, such as hiking or tennis. The purpose and type of periodized training is dependent on the individual, goals, and assessment. Take these factors, match them with the best available research, and an exercise specialist will develop a safe periodized exercise program for the nonathlete.

For example, an older adult may want to train to improve her golf game while staying healthy. The peak season for golf in South Florida is winter. Therefore, an exercise specialist can adapt the exercise program to maximize strength and endurance over the summer, while focusing on maintaining fitness and preventing injury during the winter. Another example would be a woman who wants to lose a few pounds and gain strength before having a second child. The client has provided the goals, and the exercise specialist can plan and adapt the exercise program's intensity to meet the client's needs while preventing injuries and preparing for the next "event" (childbirth). This demonstrates how credible exercise organizations and periodized plans focus on exercise specificity. Specificity is matching the exact exercise and dose to meet a person's specific goals or needs. X-Company's approach is to simply do random forms of exercise to increase "overall general physical preparedness." This concept is flawed as our body's physiology specifically adapts to the exercise and type of stresses applied – a concept of Wolff's Law is a great example of this specificity. People who do X-Company may have a difficult time carrying-over gains into another sport, particularly if certain movement patterns are not addressed. Several exercise experts voice their concerns about X-Company's heavy emphasis on exercise in only one plane (sagittal plane). Of course, the way to fix this is to simply "throw-in" different movement planes like twisting and sidebending, as X-Company's programming is completely random. The planning and preparation of a periodized training program in which exercise intensity and volume change over time produce great results for many populations. The model works, so why do we need X-Company? Has X-Company completely ignored periodized exercise training? X-Company certainly has begun heavy marketing to all populations. As evidenced in prior chapters, this expansion into new markets has come possibly without proper education, training, and proven safety. The exercise delivery of highly intense, constantly varied group exercise does not work for all populations. It is evident in several of the workouts of the day (WODs) that X-Company exercisers perform what is called AMRAP (as many repetitions as possible). How can any trainers, let alone exercisers, continually track their volume of exercise if they simply do as many movements as they can? The answer is that you don't track your volume—this would be too resonant of "traditional exercise models." It should be added that the AMRAP concept results in people pushing themselves too far, possibly resulting in lifting with bad form. Many WODs also stipulate that certain movements must be done within time limitations. For instance, perform ten pull-ups, twenty push-ups, and fifty sit-ups within seven minutes. While the purpose of a time limitation may be for working on speed, it can certainly promote a person to "rush" his or her workout to beat the clock. These techniques can be dangerous and challenging in monitoring volume and form.

Changing the sequence of when exercises are done during a workout can also change the difficulty of a workout. For instance, if an exerciser performs weight-training exercises for the legs prior to running, he will notice that the run is much more challenging than if he had simply rested before his run. The NSCA provides guidelines for the sequence of exercises in Essentials of Strength Training and Conditioning, which is cited in other chapters of this book. The NSCA promotes riskier and complex movements before other safer and more controlled exercises.

The APTA also promotes the concept of exercise sequencing based on motor control principles within an exercise as to maximize the functional potential for a client during a session (Anne Shumway-Cook and Marjorie Woollacott. Motor Control: Translating Research Into Clinical Practice. 2012: Lippincott Williams & Wilkins). For example, it is advised to perform an explosive clean and jerk prior to performing a maximum number of body-weight squats. In this example, the squats may fatigue essential muscles for stabilizing the hips and back, which may increase the risk of injury during the more challenging clean and jerk. Moreover, the maximum number of squats may reduce the weight-lifting performance of the person's clean and jerk—lifting less is obviously something a competitive athlete does not want. The practicality of these proven guidelines makes sense—X-Company simply ignores these guidelines by providing exercises in any given sequence. Many WODs include only two or three exercises done over and over again for a given time. In this cyclical fashion, a more basic exercise may be done both before and after a more complex movement several times—this greatly increases the risk for injury and overtraining. Sequencing of exercise during a workout is important; however, over the course of an exercise program, monitoring the day-to-day and week-to-week changes can be even more important.

Periodized training has been shown to be safe and effective for a multitude of populations, while providing an intense and varied program. X-Company is not needed, but people will still want to try it and success stories will continue to pour out from its marketing campaigns. If the description of the intensity of the exercise program does not raise your concerns, then perhaps an examination of the actual moves done during X-Company will shock you. Reach for the Olympic bar, grip tightly, and hold on for some X-Company movements.

IN SUMMARY:

- Rhabdo, or Uncle Rhabdo in X-Company lingo, is a serious medical condition that can occur in both fit and unfit populations.

- Rhabdo is the severe breakdown of muscle tissue, which results in kidney failure, heart irregularities, severe fatigue, and possibly death.

- X-Company is only now, after copious media exposure, addressing rhabdo by educating its staff.

- X-Company attempts to "scale" exercise to prevent injury and get the best exercise.

- Scaling is not the same as prescribing exercise or periodization, both of which are measureable and planned and can be repeated safely.

- If you are considering X-Company, try a periodized exercise program with a personal trainer or strength coach first.

- AMRAP (as many reps as possible) is very dangerous and focuses on the number of times a weight is lifted versus the form—this greatly increases your odds of injury.

- WOD (the workout of the day) may not be appropriate for your specific needs, whether it is too much weight or simply the wrong movement pattern—you can get injured.

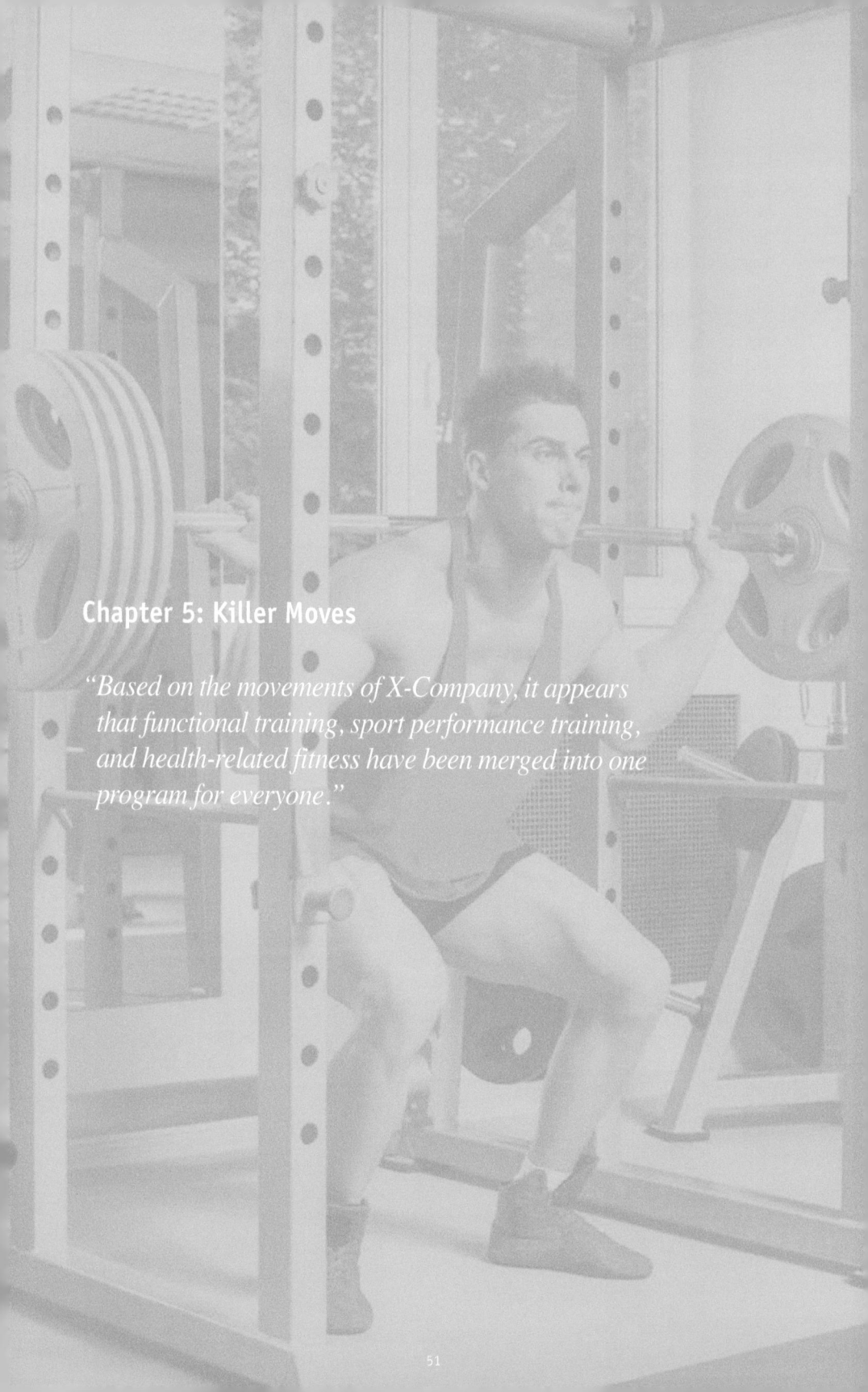

Chapter 5: Killer Moves

"Based on the movements of X-Company, it appears that functional training, sport performance training, and health-related fitness have been merged into one program for everyone."

Exercise comes in so many forms. From stretching, strengthening, neuromuscular, to sports training, exercise has such a significant impact on so many people. Our country, along with many other western nations, has seen exercise fads come and go. Be it a cause of capitalism, a desire for superficial niceties, or simply following the herd—exercise reaches billions of people each year. The moves can be simple such as body-weight exercises done at home or a basic stretching course at your local wellness center. On the other hand, the movements can be complex and intense much like X-Company and P90X®. In this chapter we will review the moves that make up X-Company.

As discussed in chapter 3, the X-Company Level 1 trainers obtain exposure to basic Olympic lifts in their Level 1 trainer's course. In the Level 2 course, the education for these Olympic lifts is further edified by requiring trainers to perform these lifts in front of other Level 2 trainers. It is apparent that these Olympic lifts form a pseudo-foundation for the X-Company staff. Moreover, with Glassman's gymnastics background, it only made sense to add gymnastic-based movements with these Olympic lifts. From a traditional exercise perspective, Olympic lifts and gymnastic movements go together like oil and water— they are designed for different sports, different movements, and different goals. Regardless, Glassman has molded these two into a nice packaged program that can be easily sold because it is unique compared to other exercise programs in the marketplace.

Greeks and Egyptians performed Olympic lifts well before Christ was born. These movements tested the physical capacity and will of these ancient men. At the time, construction methods were crude and little mechanization existed to assist with daily tasks. As such, you were highly valued if you could perform large movement patterns involving nearly the entire body with heavy loads. Having this capacity meant that you could be independent in your daily tasks, maintain your property, work, and, more importantly, defend yourself and your family. It is obvious that the Greeks and Egyptians became entrenched in many battles over the millennia, but the Olympic lifts continued through the ages only to resurge in the nineteenth century.

Many of the movements and sports that were performed in ancient times are continued today in our modern Olympics and in our field of exercise science. The competitive Olympic lifts today consist of two movements: the snatch and the clean and jerk. Lifters also perform other movements to train for these competitive Olympic lifts, such as squats, push presses, and deadlifts. It's okay if these names make no sense to you. You may not be an elite athlete, a former Greco-Roman wrestler, or a X-Company exercisers, so much of this may seem like it is Greek. So let's break down several of these movements and understand when and how they are appropriate.

X-Company is correct in saying that the squat is a foundational movement for many functional movements. From transferring to picking things up off the ground, the squat move is an essential training movement to. The squat can be prescribed for various reasons:

to improve lower body speed (U. Wisløff et al. "Strong correlation of maximal squat strength with sprint performance and vertical jump height in elite soccer players." British Journal of Sports Medicine 38.3 [2004]: 285–288), to increase lower body endurance (R. C. Hickson et al. "Potential for strength and endurance training to amplify endurance performance." Journal of Applied Physiology 65.5 [1988]: 2285–2290), to decrease the risk of falling (Stephen R. Lord et al. "The effect of an individualized fall prevention program on fall risk and falls in older people: a randomized, controlled trial." Journal of the American Geriatrics Society 53.8 [2005]: 1296–1304), and so on. The frequency, intensity, and rest time for the exercise shape how the squat will improve your health and performance. X-Company utilizes the squat in many of the movements with variable frequencies, intensities, and rest times for each workout. In theory the purpose of this variability is to prepare you for any challenge. However, research supports the idea that training at a set frequency, intensity, and rest time for several weeks to months will best facilitate a person's reaching an intended goal. Moreover, having a prescriptive approach for a period of time results in desired physiological changes— this means your body adapts to how you want it to be.

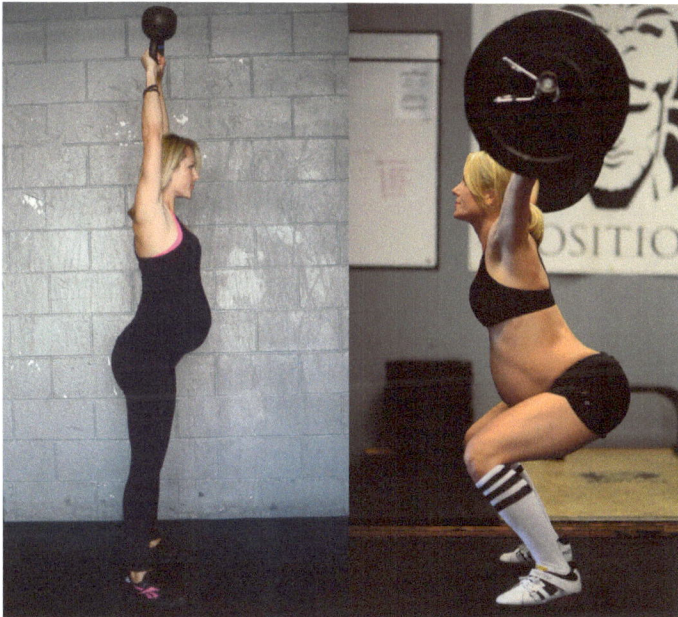

The ending position of jerk (left) and (right) snatch Olympic lifts
Permission to use by Wenn Inc.

For instance, if you are trying to perform squats to become a faster sprinter, you should perform higher intensity squats with significant rest time for recovery between sets (C. Bret et al. "Leg strength and stiffness as ability factors in 100 m sprint running." Journal of Sports Medicine and Physical Fitness 42.3 [2002]: 274–281). Given these factors, a sprinter will see her sprint become faster and her muscles transition from slower muscle fibers to faster muscle fibers (faster is better in this case). Obviously these parameters are generalized, as we are not citing a specific assessed sprinter. The use of squats is a great thing in

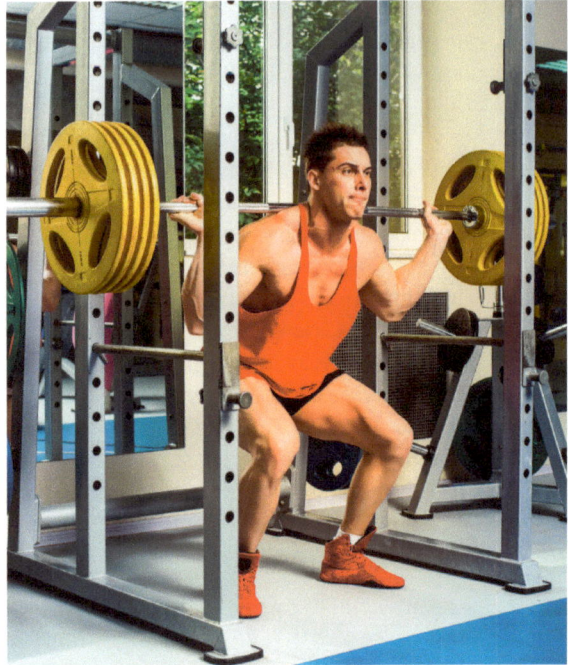

The squat
(courtesy of Shutterstock)

X-Company—I think the larger issue is the lack of prescription and training goal(s) for the squats for X-Company exercisers.

Now, imagine taking an Olympic bar from your chest and pushing it straight over your head—this is called a push press. The push press is predominately an upper-body movement. The lower body contributes to some momentum of the upward movement of the bar, while the trunk provides substantial stabilization of the spine. The movement places a significant amount of force on the shoulders, lower back, and neck. In isolation, the movement can train a person to generate significant upper-body strength and power. It can also teach a person how to combine lower-body movement with an upper-body task by the use of momentum. The concept of the push press will be further expanded as we tackle our next movement, the snatch.

The snatch is an explosive movement that taxes the entire body. In one smooth motion an Olympic barbell goes from resting on the floor to over your head with your arms fully straight. The lower body begins the movement by bringing the weight from the floor to about the height of your midthigh. At the midthigh point, the lifter explosively flings the weight overhead, placing extreme forces on the neck and shoulders. The snatch is basically

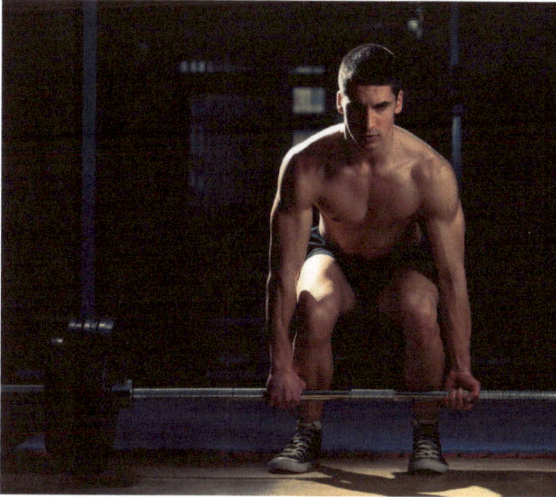

Starting position for the snatch
(courtesy of Shutterstock)

a push press only you must lift the weight from the floor and take it straight overhead. To keep things simple, we will examine the mechanics of the push press along with upper portion of the snatch movement, but be aware that these are two distinct exercises with distinctly different challenges.

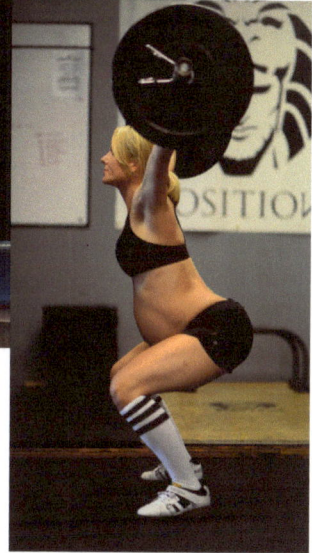

Ending position for the snatch
Permission to use by Wenn Inc.

During both the snatch, and to some degree during the push press, the risk of dropping the barbell on oneself is very high among the untrained and those not following a safe exercise progression. Having an exercise progression that includes too many of these jerks or push presses in a row, especially when coupled with other overhead exercises, can significantly increase the risk of shoulder injuries such as rotator cuff tears. The traditional purpose of the snatch and push press exercises are for power training, which includes training at lower repetitions, lots of rest, high weights, and fast movements. X-Company frequently incorporates the jerk and push press in its WODs with low weights, high repetitions, fast movements, and little rest between other exercises. Couple higher numbers of repetitions with little change in intensity day after day and this can be a recipe for what is known as a repetitive use injury (RUI).

RUIs can be in the form of calf strains, tendonitis, rotator cuff tears, and lower-back strains—these are the most common injuries in X-Company, based on interviews I have had with X-Company exercisers (recall, X-Company does not submit its injury reports to peer-reviewed journals or an injury surveillance program like NCAA has). To be fair X-Company is consistent with being variable, so there are some days X-Company exercisers do train with heavier weights and fewer repetitions in these movements. Regardless, this variable approach with an exercise such as the jerk reinforces how X-Company lacks the appropriate planning toward an individual's goal—it also lacks the control and measurability for safe exercise progression. A potential gain is available under the best conditions and preparation. The snatch and push press are fabulous lifts—leave them in the Olympics with the pros, not in the X-Company boxes with the masses.

Gymnastic Moves

Common gymnastic exercises in X-Company include movements done on rings, parallel/pull-up bars, and the open floor. A large majority of these movements are complex movements that incorporate most regions of the body. Several of the movements involve advanced coordination of multiple areas of the body at one time. The movements require athletic-level strength, stable joints, and the fortitude for heights. Let's break down some of the common gymnastic movements seen in several WODs on the rings, parallel/pull-up bars, and the open floor.

Exercises on the Rings

If you have never seen the rings on the Olympics, then imagine two large ropes hanging from a ceiling with a nine-inch diameter ring at the bottom of each rope. The rings hang approximately nine feet from the floor; as such, it usually requires a jump and a boost from a trainer in order to grab the rings. X-Company utilizes the rings to perform exercises such as dips, muscle ups, and reverse kips. Let's look at each of these movements and see what they can do for you.

A dip exercise begins with the X-Company exercisers holding the rings while his elbows are bent to more than right angle. Contracting the arm and chest muscles begins the movement up as the elbows reach full straightening. The core muscles must fire in order to prevent swaying and movement. The muscle up requires significant upper-

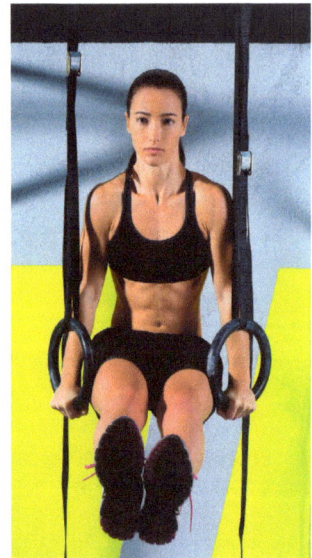

Top Portion of Muscle up
(courtesy of Shutterstock)

body and core strength. Moreover, it is very taxing on the shoulder joints and wrists. The stress on the front part of the shoulder is tremendous, especially at the lowest part of this movement. People who have had shoulder dislocations may not be able to perform this movement as they will likely dislocate their shoulders, particularly if your X-Company trainer has not done a thorough pre-exercise screening.

A muscle up is a combined movement of a pull-up and a dip. The person first starts by pull the rings to the chest. He then pulls the rings to the side of his hips, extending his elbow fully. The X-Company exerciser then lowers himself back to the starting position, which is where both arms are fully extended overhead. The muscle up exercise requires even more upper-body and core strength than the dip, as two movements are compounded into one exercise. The overhead movement and the stretching while contracting (eccentric movement) coming down can put the shoulder at risk for a cartilage (labrum) or rotator cuff tear of the shoulder, particularly if done in a ballistic fashion.

A reverse kip is an advanced movement that involves upper-body strength, core mobility, coordination, and the mental strength to not to be afraid about falling on your head. The movement begins with the X-Company exerciser pulling herself up by performing a muscle up on the rings. From this position she brings her knees to her chest and begins to allow her head and trunk to move backward. Her hands act as a fulcrum point as she performs a roll. Her hands and wrist are placed in a special grip (false grip) in order to facilitate the rolling motion. If this seems complex to understand, imagine a person holding onto rings and doing a backflip with her knees tucked. The movement is usually very controlled, but the risk of falling onto your neck or head is extremely high. I question whether the X-Company model of group exercise can ensure safety with an exercise such as the reverse kip. Moreover, the movement of rolling puts extreme stress on the wrist, despite the false grip, which can lead to ligament sprains.

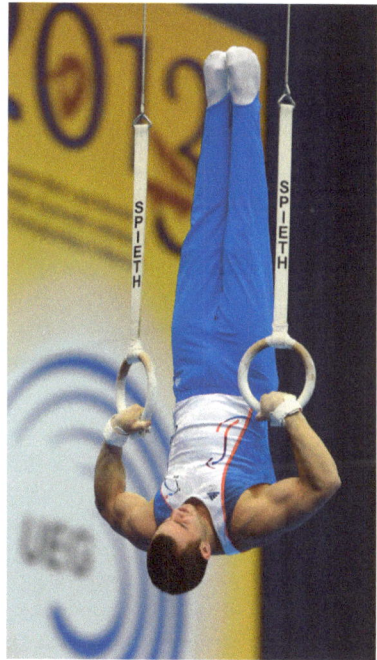

Reverse Kip
(courtesy of Shutterstock)

Exercises on the Parallel and Pull-Up Bars

Movements performed on the parallel/pull-up bars include the famous kipping pull-ups and various forms of dips and swings. If you recall your days of performing pull-ups for the Presidential Fitness Test in school, then you will remember how your coach reminded you that the pull-up was to be done with controlled movement and no leg swinging. The kipping pull-ups counter the coach's rules. X-Company's version of the pull-up involves ballistic movements that incorporate significant leg movement (swinging). It is this ballistic movement that results in a thrusting of the chest toward the bar, followed by a violent downward movement back to the starting position. Due to the large contribution from lower-body momentum, the kipping pull-up allows you to perform more "pull-ups" than would in the traditional fashion. The violent movements, particularly in an untrained person, place the shoulder and spine at great risk. In an online forum called Catalyst, several soldiers involved in military health care commented on the sharp increase in shoulder problems after X-Company began training on base (http://www.catalystathletics.com/forum/archive/index.php?t-5888-p-5.html). Their biggest concern was the pull-up and the fact they could barely move their arms for the next week after X-Company. Several studies, including one specifically involving elite military personnel, showed that high repetitions of traditional pull-ups should be avoided to prevent injury (T. W. Pelham, , L. E. Holt, and H. White. "Physical training of combat diving candidates: Implications for the prevention of musculoskeletal injuries." Work 30.4 [2008]: 423–431). The kipping pull-up increases not only the force of contraction but also the number of pull-ups done. Based on this research, the risk of shoulder injuries greatly increases, especially due to the higher forces involved in the kipping versus traditional pull-up.

Floor Exercises

X-Company exercisers also perform gymnastic moves on the "floor" which is open space within the box. These areas can be lightly padded or not at all. In these areas, several common movements can be seen. We will examine the handstand push-up and the kettlebell swing.

The handstand push-up is fairly self-explanatory. A person may guide you into a handstand position. If you have no buddy or trainer, a wall or piece of equipment is used to help maintain your balance at your feet, which are in the air. The X-Company exerciser then performs push-ups in this handstand position by bending his elbows and shoulders. Several progressions evolve from this exercise including walking on your hands and walking with push-ups. X-Company prides itself in designing a program focused on functioning. How does walking or performing push-ups in a handstand position carry over to any functional move? Outside of being a gymnast, which few of us are, this exercise puts the general population at great risk of injury to the head and neck. Furthermore, several authors have published the risk of overhead activity and its impact on the rotator cuff and ligaments of the shoulder (P. A. Borsa, K. G. Laudner, and E. L. Sauers. "Mobility and stability adaptations in the shoulder of the overhead athlete: A theoretical and evidence-based perspective." Sports Medicine 38.1 [2008]: 17–36). These authors argue that repetitive overhead movements can increase the chance of rotator cuff tears. Plain and simple: handstand exercises are not safe unless you are a trained gymnast with a specific sports training program, and even then there is still a risk for injury.

Another exercise commonly performed on the floor is the kettlebell swing. A kettlebell is a large, usually heavy (thirty-five pounds and up) weight with a large handle shaped like the handle of tea kettle. Kettlebells allow exercisers to perform movements different than what traditional dumbbells offer. In the case of a kettlebell swing they allow a X-Company exerciser to grab the weight from the handle and swing it repeatedly overhead. The exercise has its merit; however, the weight is usually so heavy that extreme trunk and lower-body power is needed to generate the momentum to swing the weight. The proper form is to not use the arms alone. As such the kettlebell swing can be dangerous if you have lower-back issues (Bryan Fass. "Injury prevention In EMS." *TSAC Report* [2013]: 15) and may cause hand injuries (Karuppaiah Karthik et al. "Extensor Pollicis Brevis tendon damage presenting as de Quervain's disease following kettlebell training." *BMC Sports Science, Medicine and Rehabilitation* 5.1 [2013]: 13). The kettlebell swing can be a challenging yet rewarding exercise, but good form and appropriate prescription to the right athlete is needed in order to avoid injury.

Gymnastic exercises provide a way for X-Company to stand out from the traditional exercise pack. It is this deviation from the norm, along with the Olympic lifts and overall exercise intensity, that make X-Company dangerous, particularly for the general population. Olympic and gymnastic movements are meant for athletes, especially at the volume of movements that X-Company exercisers desire to complete. X-Company movements are overly repetitive, place several joints at their breaking points, and are sometimes questionable as to their functional need (e.g., handstand walking). Based on the movements of X-Company, it appears that functional training, sport performance training, and health-related fitness have been merged into one program for everyone.

Health, Functional, and Sports Performance Training

The exercise and rehabilitation world has kept things nicely organized over the last several decades. Health-related fitness training provides a person a way to improve his or her heart health, lose some weight, or gain strength for activities. Health-related fitness programs are safe, prescribed individually, progressive, and often include movements with varied pieces of exercise equipment. Research has shown the effectiveness and safety of health-related fitness for several populations (Jaana H. Suni et al. "Safety and feasibility of a health-related fitness test battery for adults." *Physical Therapy* 78.2 [1998]: 134–148).

Functional training has its roles in several populations. From helping elderly adults to be able to more safely rise from a chair to a soldier being able to ascend a wall, functional training is designed to be specific to a person's life or job functions. The training is movement specific: it closely mimics what that person needs to be doing without actually doing that function. The intensity is specific to the intensity of the movement, but form always trumps intensity because injuries can occur. The NSCA and APTA advocate that if functional training cannot be performed safely, more basic exercises need to be implemented, such as traditional weight training or controlled exercises that are not functional.

Sports performance training has been classically defined as exercise training that is specific to a sport, and it usually is centered on a periodized training program. Sports performance training includes traditional weight lifting, power lifting, and conditioning exercises with functional (sport functions) training. Intensity is variable but planned and closely monitored. Certified strength and conditioning specialists (CSCSs) are truly experts in this arena of training.

In the development of a new trend, X-Company has dumped the traditional health-related fitness program concepts. With it went the safety precautions and screenings as discussed in chapter 3. Traditional weight training and conditioning exercise has been forced out of the X-Company training programming. Moreover, given that X-Company attempts to prepare its followers for "generalized physical preparedness," it has ignored the concept of sport performance training. Apparently only CSCSs have time for periodized training programs and to closely monitor exercise volume and intensity. X-Company has a functional training bias with inherent disregard of health-related measures and exercise intensity/volume.

The movements in X-Company are supposed to be "functional." I questioned the handstand push-ups; however, what about the other movements? When would a thirty-year-old woman have to perform a kettlebell swing at her office? Perhaps she would do this movement if her monitor died and she was very angry, slinging the monitor into the air. When would a fifty-year-old golfer need to climb a rope? Maybe if he lost a ball in a tree and he luckily found a tire swing to gain access to the canopy of that tree. When would person need to perform a kip tuck roll on parallel bars? You can see the absurdity in analyzing the movement with daily physical needs.

The notion that the movements in X-Company are purely "functional" is a complete farce. Granted, these movements may be functional for some groups (e.g., soldiers, gymnasts, athletes, etc.), but they are not appropriate for a large majority of the population. The notion that these movements can be done by anyone defeats the actual intended purpose of functional training. Recall, functional training programs help people perform a functional task that is needed. If someone does not need to climb a rope or flip themselves on bars in daily life, why are these movements part of their exercise program? I cannot recall the last time I needed to perform a 150-pound overhead press in my daily activity—even as a personal trainer. An exercise expert creates a functional training program to meet an individual's activity or sporting needs. The individual's activity or sporting needs are not best met by a generalized, pseudo-functional training program with constantly variable metrics. The lack of specificity for individuals' performance goals is glaringly apparent within X-Company.

Perhaps the next evolution for X-Company will be gyms and businesses that spin off as "X-Company Lite" or "Periodized X-Company Training." Only time will tell the evolution of X-Company and its moves. X-Company attempts to prepare a person for any physical challenge—but at what cost?

IN SUMMARY, X-COMPANY MOVEMENTS:

- Are a combination of Olympic lifts, gymnastic movements, and other "functional moves"

- Include Olympic lifts and variants of these movements: snatch, clean and jerk, squat, and deadlifts

- Can be done on rings, parallel/pull-up bars, or the open floor

- Can have you performing an Olympic lift, a gymnastic ring exercise, and a functional rope movement all in the same workout

- Are likely to increase joint and muscle injuries, as many of the movements promote extreme ranges of motion and forceful contractions, even when a person is fatigued

- Are claimed to be functional, although few actually carry over into normal daily living

- Are disconnected from individuals' specific performance goals and functioning

- Are combined health, functional, and sports-performance training

Chapter 6: Special Populations

"Guidelines for Exercise and Kids: too much, too quick, with lacking supervision can result in injury."

We have covered several major parameters of exercise (e.g., the moves, intensity, prescription, etc.). It should be apparent that exercise can be for everyone. The intended purpose of exercise is dependent on a person's goals, health status, and psyche. A well-trained, educated, and contemporary exercise specialist designs a program for each person's needs and limitations. An individualized exercise approach is especially important for those people with physical, mental, or medical limitations—these "special populations" need special attention that X-Company cannot offer.

What About the Children?

I introduced the concept of X-Company Kids when discussing the educational competencies of X-Company trainers. The X-Company Kids program has good intentions: get our youth moving. However, X-Company Inc. has not considered the major exercise and health ramifications at stake for these little ones.

The box was surprisingly full of teenagers during my X-Company assessment. The teenagers seemed to keep good pace with the posted WOD; unfortunately I did see one thirteen-year-old girl injure her knee at the very beginning of the workout. The head trainer offered no assessment but did provide her a bag of ice. I thought to myself: What happened to her knee? Will she continue X-Company? What kind of damage might be done (and may continue to happen)? Will her parents wonder what happened and whether it is safe?

Several parents have asked me if it is safe for their six-year-old son to lift weights? Or they might ask how much running is okay for their ten-year-old daughter? Before 2008, the field of medicine had a dearth of knowledge regarding such questions, leaving some fitness specialists, including X-Company trainers, to simple conjecture.

In 2008 the American College of Sports Medicine published the "Physical Activity Guidelines for Americans." In these guidelines, researchers revealed that exercise is essential not only for most Americans but especially children. With obesity, bone loss, and heart disease a concern, the authors of the guidelines advise children to participate in at least sixty minutes of moderate to vigorous exercise each day. The growing demands of extracurricular activities, the rigors of schoolwork, and the stress of two working parents all seem to be barriers for these children to engage in physical activity. The authors cited that exercise specialists, researchers, and parents have traditionally seen cardiovascular exercise, such as swimming and biking, as safe for children. The authors further stated that weight training for children is a safe and an effective way to build muscles, burn calories, and strengthen bones. Here are some additional principles from the guidelines:

- The risk of injury with weight training is no greater than that seen in common sports.

- Kids do not need testosterone to gain strength or muscle mass.

- Growth plate fractures have never been reported in programs supervised and safely designed by exercise specialists. Kids' growth or height will not be stunted—if anything, exercise will be supportive to normal development.

- The guidelines recommend that exercise specialists follow established training guidelines to reduce risk of injury.

Herein lies the rub: X-Company trainers do not follow established training guidelines. Recall, they have created their own workout routine, without published research, that runs counter to many of the established exercise principles. In short, X-Company is not meeting the ACSM's guidelines for properly training children.

Does X-Company follow the NSCA's "Position Statement for Youth Resistance Training"? To weed through some of the banal research jargon, I have summarized the findings from this publication:

- A properly designed and supervised program can improve these factors in youth: strength, power, physiologic status, motor skill performance, and psychosocial well-being

- A properly designed and supervised program can reduce the risk of cardiovascular disease in youth

- A properly designed and supervised program can promote and develop exercise habits (e.g., kids that exercise will likely continue to exercise into their teens) in youth

- A properly designed and supervised program is relatively safe for youth

The iterative theme is apparent: a properly designed and supervised program. The NSCA's findings are consistent with the ACSM's findings for youth exercise. X-Company does not offer a structured and or developmentally proper design to its kids' program; as such, the program does not meet the standards of the NSCA.

In the NSCA's position statement, the authors find that adolescent athletes had higher rates of injury related to resistance training when aggressive progression of training loads or improper exercise had been used. **X-Company proudly holds the honors for one of the most aggressive exercise programs in the marketplace**. Recall that X-Company trainers do not track exercise volume or periodize their training programs. Moreover, the volume and repetitions of the exercise can be such that X-Company exercisers often finish their sets with poor form. As such, the exercise implemented in X-Company can be considered both "improper" and aggressive—both of which increase the risk of injury in adolescent athletes.

Supervision during X-Company training is done through group exercise. The method of group exercise has been shown to be effective for other youth and adolescent sports and physical activity programs. As such, the issue with the X-Company Kids program is the lack of exercise program design and planning, which is considered best practice standards by the NSCA.

If these guidelines and position statements are not sufficient evidence for my concern with X-Company Kids, let's examine what another expert has to say. During an ABC interview, Dr. Paul Stricker, a pediatric sports medicine specialist, provided ample expert opinion evidence that X-Company may be very risky for youth (http://abcnews.go.com/blogs/health/2013/11/06/is-crossfit-training-safe-for-children/). He repeats much of what was covered in the NSCA and ACSM guidelines: too much, too quick, with lacking supervision can result in injury. In the interview, the X-Company Kids representative saw it differently, stating, "Our intention is to make children safer in their daily lives, such as when lifting a backpack or on the field of play when they have to run, cut, jump, etc." The intentions of X-Company Kids seem altruistic and original. But keep in mind that X-Company is a business and that exercise specialists have been providing these exact services years before X-Company trainers started.

The Coach and Life Coaches

If you are thirty years or older, think back to your days in elementary or middle school. The best period or block of time was likely during physical education (unless you did not have physical prowess or feared the changing of clothes before and after "gym class" in front of your peers). Physical education, or PE, offered you the opportunity to run, play, and formulate teams for competitive sports. I asked those who were thirty years or older to think back nostalgically for a reason—many twenty-year-olds and teenagers have missed PE altogether.

According to the National Association of Sport and Physical Education (NASPE), only about half of students nationwide are enrolled in physical education (http://www.aahperd.org/naspe/standards/nationalGuidelines/PAguidelines.cfm). The numbers get worse as students get older: nearly one-third of high school students actively take a physical education course. As students exercise less, researchers are finding the rates for obesity are climbing.

The Centers for Disease Control and Prevention (CDC) reported in January 2012 that nearly 17 percent of children (two to nineteen years old) were obese. The largest proportion, about 20 percent, of obese children were boys from six to nineteen years old. Meanwhile, only 14.4 percent of boys from two to five years old ("preschoolers") were obese. Simply examining these data, one can see the possible effect the academic system may have on our children (http://www.cdc.gov/nchs/data/databriefs/db82.pdf).

Figure 2. Prevalence of obesity among children and adolescents aged 2–19, by sex and age: United States, 2009–2010

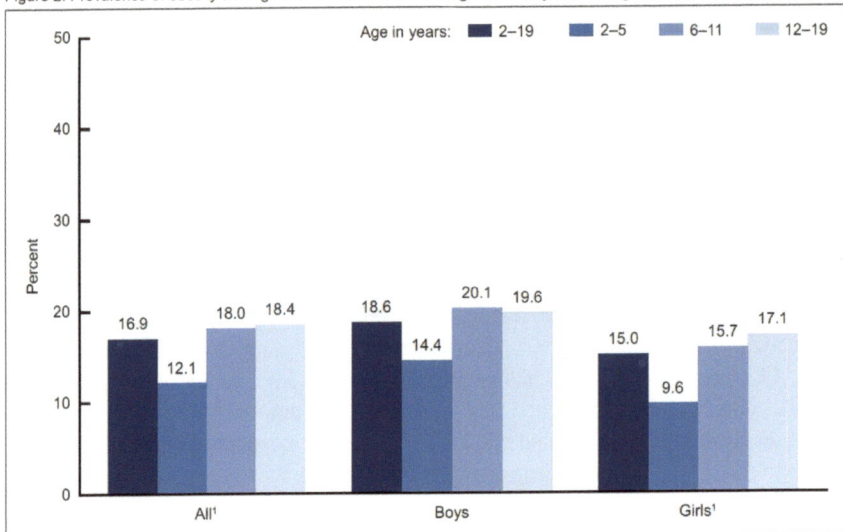

Age in years: ■ 2–19   ■ 2–5   ■ 6–11   ▢ 12–19

[1]Significant increasing linear trend by age ($p < 0.005$).
SOURCE: CDC/NCHS, National Health and Nutrition Examination Survey, 2009–2010.

Figure: Graph of Obesity Prevalence Among Children

Journalists and reporters across the country continue to write about how schools are transitioning time away from physical education to more time in the classroom. Standardized testing, funding calculations for schools, and student pressure to enroll into college seem to be the big drivers in the transition from exercise to more book time. Moreover, other data support that students not enrolled in physical education during school do not make up the exercise time outside of school.

I never realized the impact of taking away physical education time until I began teaching undergraduate students in 2009. The class I was teaching was a foundational exercise course for exercise science students. The average age in the class was twenty.

I assigned my students a small hands-on examination based on a case scenario. The case scenario involved different mock athletes or clients who needed different exercise selections. The students were to select one exercise and perform that exercise with me as their "client." Several professors thought the concept was a bit advanced for such novice students; however, I had covered beyond the textbook and was willing to be lenient in grading as long as students covered some core concepts outlined in my objectives.

One of the prompts I provided the students included a first baseman who wanted to improve his reach to catch a ball when thrown at him. In the prompt, the first baseman reported tightness in his inner thigh that was impeding his stretch to catch the ball. I chose this scenario as it seemed very straightforward and students would easily match the exercise with the client's need.

As the day of examinations progressed, I began to notice a trend. Almost half of the students who randomly selected the first baseman scenario struggled. At first I thought that the scenario had been too complex. Next, I considered that the students might have simply been nervous, particularly since this was an "athlete." Students did not get heavy exposure to athletes in this course, but this particular concept would apply to athletes or nonathletes. To get to the root of the issue, I pulled the handful of students aside and spoke with them individually. Needless to say, I was flabbergasted to find that these students did not know what a first baseman was.

The national pastime of baseball had become nonexistent to portion of my class. How did this happen? Two of the students remarked that they never had played this sport in school—whether in PE or for a club team. The other student had no interest in exercise, health, or sport; as such, she never bothered to explore these concepts in PE or within her circle of friends. The other student had heard of the sport but had no concept of how it was played. How can children live nearly two decades and not understand the legendary sport of baseball? It is easy to see how altering kids' physical education courses have already had a negative impact. Albeit these students comprised a small percentage of the class (15 to 20 percent) I had, but I would argue that all students twenty years ago could have easily understood the basic fundamentals of baseball—especially naming the function of the man who stands on the first of four bases. Some X-Company exercisers ask how does an X-Company exerciser differ than a PE Coach – the answer is usually a bachelor's degree and the emphasis on less-intense, lifelong exercise and activity. Furthermore, X-Company advertises and promotes itself as a sport – not a class built into our educational system. As a "sport," shouldn't they follow similar exercise guidelines as those in the NCAA and professional leagues?

The educational system in America needs reform. The funding, politicians, and parents need a paradigm shift. In an attempt to not digress too far from the topic of this book, I will be succinct: our educational system is slowly failing our kids in teaching them how to exercise and stay active. If you need a solution for obesity, start in the schools where students are not moving but slices of pizza are flying off the shelves.

The answer comes about with responsible adults making responsible decisions. It starts from the top, with community leaders ensuring we instill that physical education is a vital component to our educational system. Science, technology, engineering, and mathematics, while important for the economy and solving world problems, does not trump the lessons learned and physiological impact gleaned while in PE. Parents should charge their leaders to make PE a priority and not simply an elective. Parents can be the key solution for society to curb our obesity and chronic health epidemic.

Despite parents leading the charge to help our children, they may need to stop and look in the mirror first. Sixty percent of adults are overweight. Thirty-five percent of adults are obese, according to the CDC in 2009 and 2010 (http://www.cdc.gov/nchs/data/databriefs/db82.pdf). The rates of chronic health conditions, such as diabetes, coronary heart disease, stroke, and hypertension, will mirror the data of obesity; as obesity trends higher, so will these diseases. Looking at this grim data, you might ask yourself, why are so many Americans obese? The answer may seem simple, but the figure may shock you. Eighty percent of American adults do not meet minimal exercise guidelines (http://www.cbsnews.com/news/cdc-80-percent-of-american-adults-dont-get-recommended-exercise/). That equates to just roughly one in five people who actually are meeting the minimal guidelines of exercise. Seeing these numbers it makes sense why so many adults are overweight or obese. Now, factor in a high-stress job or school, the perception of limited time, family responsibilities, and a poor diet: you have the grand recipe for not just a few pounds but several chronic diseases. How can these 80 percent of Americans lead our children to health?

The answer is a tough one to swallow—parents may not be the best role model based on the data. However, knowing parents and having seen the transformation in my own patients, I am certain parents can lead their both their children and themselves into a healthier future. The steps begin with simple measures of reducing sitting time, increasing activity, and focus on exercising:

- One of the easiest cures is to cancel the cable subscription and remove any streaming video devices. You will suddenly notice you have an extra hour or two of available time to play in the yard, walk to the playground, or ride a bike with your child.

- If you feel intimidated by a gym or think you are out of shape, start with simple unstructured physical activity. Walk to your neighbor's house or the grocery store. Bike with your daughter to the playground. Use nonmechanized forms of transportation to get from one location to another. Don't focus on the time or intensity—just begin moving.

- If after you start moving you feel prepared to advance your activity, then consider joining a local wellness center. Take your family or meet after work and school for a family workout. If machines seem boring, consider taking a group exercise class of boxing or dancing. Racquetball courts are also a great way to smash out some frustration while requiring little expertise to play.

Making the Move to Getting Them Moving

As parents become more active, so will their children. I can say that I am happy to see X-Company is making the move to getting adults and children to exercise. With the given data and continued trends of poor health, it would seem that any exercise may be good. But this may be only half true.

Muscle soreness is a common complaint from people who begin to exercise. It is this muscle soreness and injures that will sideline and discourage many from continuing to exercise. An appropriately assessed, prescribed, and progressive exercise program will ease a client into exercise, while preventing injury. The information provided in the prior chapters sheds light into the many mechanisms of injury from X-Company. As such, X-Company is not the exercise of choice to get the masses, whether it is children or adults, moving for a lifetime.

IN SUMMARY:

- X-Company Kids does not meet ACSM or NSCA exercise guidelines for children or adolescents.

- According to a leading expert, X-Company Kids may increase the risk of injury for your child.

- Children are losing exercise and physical activity time in and out of school.

- A majority of American adults are not meeting minimal exercise guidelines.

- Chronic diseases, such as obesity and heart disease, continue to climb in the United States.

- Exercise and health education are vital to making our country healthy.

- X-Company is not the best option for getting people to move and improving health without risking injury.

Chapter 7: A Cross in the Road: X-Company's Future

"X-Company's recent rhabdo and stress-urinary incontinence issues have drawn strong criticism from physical therapists and fitness specialists. What's next?"

X-Company has exploded in worldwide popularity. In prior chapters we covered X-Company's culture, educational competencies, and training parameters. X-Company's media contract, games, and expansion into commercialized products show that X-Company shows no signs of slowing down. What is next for X-Company?

The biggest push has been to expand its range of clientele. The leaders of X-Company understand that young, healthy post-college-age professionals are their bread and butter. Maintaining the flow of these individuals into boxes is a must. But what about other populations: the high school teenagers, the middle-aged office personnel, and the aged? X-Company's management knows that these are the people who improve their bottom line; as such, the X-Company marketing for these populations have exploded in the last five years. With marketing hooks such as "It Is for All People, Shapes, and Sizes" and "Think You're Too Old or X-Company Is Too Hard?" it is easy to see how X-Company and its affiliates are targeting a diversified group of people. (http://www.prevention.com/fitness/strength-training/crossfit-women-over-50canX-Company, http://www.X-Companyatlanta.com/X-Company_atlanta/too-hard.html).

The ABC News story regarding X-Company's expansion into X-Company Kids supports the position that X-Company is purposively expanding into new markets. In chapter 3 you read that the X-Company trainer is not educated to work with such a population. Moreover, in chapter 6 you noted that the intensity and frequency of X-Company training could damage an adolescent's body. Yet X-Company Inc. plows forward expanding into new markets in search of new business.

Greg Glassman, the owner of X-Company Inc., knows he has gotten big—so big that it is hard to rein in gyms that offer "X-Company-type" training that do not hold X-Company licensing and certification agreements. X-Company's management boasts a strong team of legal professionals that aggressively pursue nonlicensed boxes and noncertified individuals offering pseudo-X-Company training. The company obviously shut down my first edition of this book, so their legal team is certainly active. Despite this, maintaining and tracking the number of these facilities and trainers can be challenging, as the fitness industry has high turnover and little regulation. These "X-Company-type" facilities see opportunity in providing a similar service at possibly a lower price. After all, what high-schooler or older adult on a fixed income can afford a monthly X-Company fee of $500?

One "X-Company-style" training business that has done well is the Iron Tribe (www.irontribefitness.com). It offers an X-Company-style of training that is less intense than X-Company at a more affordable price. Less-intense X-Company is appealing to those with medical issues and the older adults. While the more affordable price is compelling for most people, it is especially of interest for those younger athletes and older adults on a fixed income. It is businesses such as Iron Tribe that may cut into X-Company's bottom line over time, as it undermines X-Company's expansion into the young, the unhealthy middle-aged, and the aged. How can X-Company compete with these facilities and continue its expansion? The answer to X-Company's survival is to win the heart and minds of other health, fitness, and medical professionals. Based on several recent scathing media exposés, few medical professionals are in glaring support of X-Company. Physicians want their patients to exercise, but as a whole, physicians tend to be very conservative about exercise and diet modifications. Whether the conservative approach to exercise and diet is appropriate or not, the fact is that most people listen and follow their physicians' orders. Moreover, X-Company's recent rhabdo and stress-urinary incontinence issues have drawn strong criticism from physical therapists and fitness specialists. Certified strength and conditioning specialists (CSCSs) from the National Strength and Conditioning Association (NSCA) also hold an informal grudge against X-Company because X-Company claims to be a "strength and conditioning program." It should be noted that CSCSs have been providing high-intensity and variable training for years, although with greater precision, planning, and sport-specificity. In short, X-Company has not fortified friends across the fitness and health community.

Perhaps the fitness industry in general needs a revamping? As we discussed earlier, the certification requirements for both X-Company and some traditional trainers can be extremely weak, with some trainers taking simple weekend or online courses and then calling themselves "health/fitness experts." The certification exams for these rogue trainers must stop. Therefore, we need a regulatory body that can force these programs to close. Perhaps part of this regulatory body could include a national, central examining board should be implemented – this ought to apply to X-Company too, especially given their weak ANSI accreditation for their exam. After trainers pass their approved examination they then can apply for a license to train in their respective state. Licensing will ensure trainers will have background checks and accountant for continuing education standards. Obviously licensing would be done state-by-state, but the overseeing national organization(s) could have input and sway into state laws and regulations for licensing. Similar organizational structures and regulations are in place in Canada and the European Union – why not America? So, for those X-Company exercisers arguing that I simply hate X-Company: I say let's make a better National Exercise System.

With the fitness industry recommendations aside, X-Company can ensure its survival and win several partners through enhancing its professional behaviors, advancing its education, and adopting health and fitness guidelines and screenings for exercise and safety. Recommendations for X-Company's future success follow in bold:

1. 1. Establish a credible professional X-Company organization that requires membership dues, institutes a code of ethics, establishes a peer-reviewed journal, and provides practice direction for its members.

a. a. A membership requirement would show that X-Company personnel care about the organization and are willing to invest in it. A membership demonstrates to the general population and health/fitness personnel that you are credible and legitimate.

2. Write and follow a Code of Ethics.

a. All major professional health and fitness organizations have codes of ethics. These ensure that their members practice and run their business ethically. Failure to meet these codes can result in disciplinary action, such as the retraction of a license or certification.

3. Establish a peer-reviewed journal.

a. A peer-reviewed journal improves the rigors of your research, which will enhance practice patterns and safety. Peer-reviewed means that you have a multidisciplinary team that reviews, edits, and publishes content relative to X-Company, exercise, and/or health. Having this team and journal eliminates bias and shows other researchers and health professionals that an organization is committed to lifetime health and wellness. Without a journal, X-Company runs the risk of other health-care providers ruining its name in other journals biased against X-Company.

i. A peer-reviewed journal will allow X-Company an avenue to publish injury trends.

4. Establish practice patterns and guidelines.

a. Establishing practice patterns and guidelines for X-Company trainers is a must. A "handbook" or "training book" is not sufficient as it is not expansive enough, nor does it teach critical thinking and analysis.

b. Demonstrate that your members can work with other health-care providers. Show that your trainers, organization, and management are willing to work with physical therapists, CSCSs, and medical doctors. The client/patient needs all health/fitness providers to work together to achieve the best care.

c. A professional organization can also accredit teaching centers/affiliate members. At this point X-Company Inc. provides generalized guidelines for its affiliate members in how to educate future trainers. *X-Company Inc. does not accredit, inspect, or measure the success of these affiliate gyms. As such, the only requirement for a box to begin and continue to educate new trainers every year is money.*

5. 5. Improve the educational competencies and establish accreditation for X-Company trainers' education.

a. The American College of Sports Medicine (ACSM), American Physical Therapy Association (APTA), and National Athletic Trainers' Association (NATA) all have standards for accreditation for educating and training exercise and rehabilitation professionals.

b. The model exists: X-Company first needs to establish its professional association and then follow similar accreditation models, such as the organizations listed above.

c. Accreditation will strengthen the education and training of the trainers, which will improve clients' performance and enhance safety.

6. Adopt the ACSM Health Risk Stratification and Screening (or similar guidelines).

a. These guidelines were discussed in chapter 3 and provide an easy way to prevent sudden death while exercising. Without some model or screening requirement, X-Company boxes will continue to accept new exercisers without appropriate screening and safety mechanisms in place.

b. Adopting these guidelines does not mean the exercise at X-Company will be "weaker"— it will simply be safer. Anyone arguing against safety while exercising has either a conflict of interest or is not educated appropriately.

7. Integrate more in-depth assessment tools directed at individualized assessment for performance and health.

a. Perform pre-exercise health screenings that at the minimum include heart rate, blood pressure, and a health history review.

b. Perform pre-exercise functional assessments to ensure that a client has the ability to perform many of the X-Company moves.

c. Perform fitness assessments; detailed guidelines for these are available from the ACSM. These assessments will allow for:

   i. Better prescription (scaling) for each client

   ii. Better measurement for success/progress in each client

d. Having more detailed screenings equates to more referrals to medical providers, when indicated.

   i. More medical referrals can provide better injury surveillance and create a positive relationship between X-Company staff and medical personnel.

These changes may seem easy to some reading these recommendations. In reality, these changes would make profound, global modifications for an exploding business model with thousands of participants. The above changes will not come easily but can be achieved. The ACSM, NATA, and APTA are all great examples of how an organization can expand while maintaining quality education, advancing research, and evolving practice patterns to best help patients.

What Now?

Whether you still are considering joining an X-Company box after reading this book or are simply interested in hiring an exercise specialist of some type, please consider the following recommendations. I have provided these in a simple tear-out version near the end of the book for you to clip out and carry with you.

Be seen by your primary care physician. Discuss beginning X-Company with him or her. Ask your physician if it is safe for you and your specific needs. If you cannot get a specific response, ask your physician what his or her hesitation may be. Physicians do not always know what is best in regards to exercise; however, they will know your medical limitations and the factors that affect your survivability in a physiologically intense program such as X-Company.

1. **Research gyms (boxes) and fitness specialists.** There are trainers and then there are trainers with advanced degrees, specializations, and multidisciplinary approaches. For instance, some trainers will also be registered nurses, physical therapists, or exercise physiologists—the additional education and credentialing make a significant difference. Eliminate from your list the "globo-gym" personal trainers and beautiful bodies that talk endlessly about their supplements and big biceps. Large gyms usually mean mediocre trainers and vague/generalized trainer backgrounds. Small to midsize gyms and especially private facilities offer more select trainers who have an intended focus, population, or specialty. In these facilities, the trainers' main role is not to wipe equipment or make a large membership upsell; instead, they are fully engaged with their clients in helping them get better.

2. **Ask for references or a résumé.** A good trainer will have a track record: what are others in the community saying about this trainer or facility? A résumé can provide a deeper look at a trainer's education (both past and recent exercise-related continuing education) and provide you with the level of engagement he or she has with the profession. In other words, does your future trainer embrace, live, and breathe exercise—or is he or she simply putting time in the gym to make a buck. Usually those who are dedicated hold active memberships in professional organizations, attend yearly conventions, and even present or publish articles. Ask if the trainer holds CPR certification and professional liability insurance. Look for a trainer with a minimum of an associate's degree in an exercise-related field (e.g., athletic training, human performance, sports medicine, kinesiology, physical therapy, or exercise science). The additional educational rigor will enhance your training experience immensely.

3. **Hold an interview and visit the facility.** Meeting the person you will be working with is essential. Confirm items you have noted from their résumé or website. Be sure to ask relevant questions that pertain to your specific goals and needs. Your future trainer ought to be able to provide solid recommendations and objective means to meet your needs—if not, ask him or her who can help you best. At the end of the day, you are engaging in a relationship for optimal health, which holds serious ramifications for your future potential and pocketbook. Inspect the facility during your meeting. It should be clean, organized,

and offer equipment for your needs (e.g., sport training equipment if you are training for football, or balance training equipment if you need help with your balance). Recall that equipment is only as good as those who are using it—too many people buy into medical and wellness fads simply because businesses advertise space-age technology. The staff delivers the care, not the equipment. Equipment should be spaced out sufficiently (e.g., three feet) to prevent collisions and tripping. Lastly, ask when the equipment was professionally inspected for mechanical faults—some facilities only clean their machines, which can put you at risk for injury.

4. **Ask for a free trial session.** Try a session before you buy. See if you, the trainer, and the facility work in unison. See if the trainer makes specific modifications for you and your needs. Examine the facility for items you may not have noticed during your first visit. The investment in your health is a serious matter—speak up if you don't feel the facility or trainer meets your needs. Committing to a center or trainer for a series of sessions can be both a financial and physical mistake that can leave both you and your wallet hurting.

5. **Periodically reassess your trainer and facility.** Has your trainer adapted your program as you have progressed? Have others training around you continued or has there been a high amount of turnover? Stable and successful facilities dedicated to their clients' goals and lifetime wellness will have long-term, satisfied clients. Centers that are focused on short-term profits and superficial training mind-sets will have a high rate of turnover. Also note whether the facility has had repairs, clean towels, and routine cleaning of equipment—several studies have shown that some forms of resistant bacteria like to grow on gym equipment handles and seats!

6. **If choosing to go with a X-Company facility:**
a. **Ensure that your trainer has performed a health screening and a functional and fitness assessment on you; this involves the trainer reviewing your health problems, asking you to perform functional movements like squatting, and assessing your strength/flexibility/and other body measures (e.g., heart rate, blood pressure, weight).**
b. **Ask that your program be "scaled" exactly to you, based on your functional and fitness assessment.**
c. **Demand that the training staff monitor or educate you on how to monitor your heart rate and appropriate response to exercise.**
i. **Consider purchasing a heart rate monitor watch with a chest strap (the brand Polar® makes excellent heart rate watches)**
d. **When in doubt: stop. Listen to your body, ask the staff to watch your form carefully, and do not get faulted into lifting more/faster/harder. Your body is a temple—take care of it by not exercising to an extreme.**
e. **If you become injured, seek licensed medical professionals (e.g., physicians, physical therapists). If routinely injured or severely injured, consider quitting X-Company and look for a better-qualified fitness specialist.**

I have a passion for educating others. Moreover, I have high standards for exercise, health, and rehabilitation. I genuinely care about my clients and patients. As such, I want the best for my clients, loved ones, and even you. I may not know you, but I am committed to helping you to achieve the best of health and empowering you to learn how to do it safely. If you have purchased or even borrowed this book from a friend, I hope that you will learn several ways to protect yourself and engage in fun exercise that is good for your body and soul!

Please follow, engage, and further the discussion with me at:

Website: www.double-crossed.com

Blog: http://DoubleCrossedBook.tumblr.com

Facebook: https://www.facebook.com/DoubleCrossedBook

Twitter: https://www.twitter.com/DoubleCrossedCF

The Six Tips to Finding the Right Trainer and Facility

Tear out this sheet to remind you of the things you need to do before and during your personal training experience.

1. Be seen by your primary care physician yearly.

2. Research gyms (boxes) and fitness specialists.

a. Focus on finding a small to midsize gym or private facility.

3. Ask for references or a résumé.

a. Ask if the trainer holds CPR certification and professional liability insurance.

b. Look for a trainer with a minimum of an associate's degree in an exercise-related field (e.g., athletic training, human performance, sports medicine, kinesiology, physical therapy, or exercise science).

4. Hold an interview and visit the facility.

a. Meet the person you will be working with and ask relevant questions that pertain to your specific goals and needs.

b. Ensure that the facility is clean, organized, and offers equipment for your needs.

c. Ask about equipment maintenance.

5. Ask for a free trial session.

6. Periodically reassess your trainer and facility.

a. Ensure that your program is adapted as you have progressed or had issues.

b. Note whether the facility has had repairs, has clean towels, and performs routine cleaning of equipment.

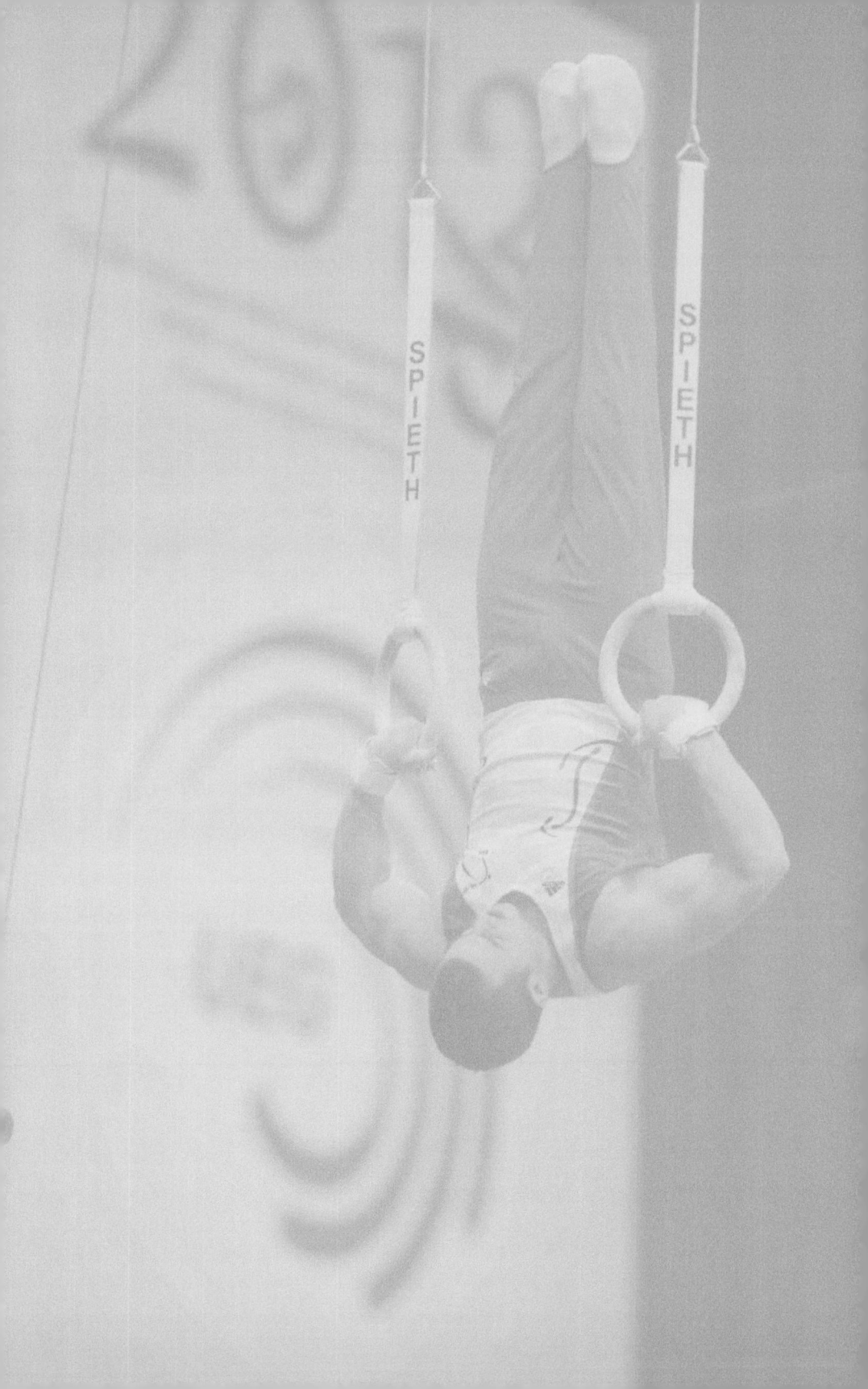